THE ENERGY RESET PLAN

6 WEEKS TO FEELING STRONGER, HEALTHIER & HAPPIER

THE ENERGY RESET PLAN

6 WEEKS
TO FEELING STRONGER, HEALTHIER & HAPPIER

ROSIE MILLEN

Nutritional Therapist

hamlyn

An Hachette UK Company
www.hachette.co.uk

First published in Great Britain in 2021
by Mitchell Beazley, an imprint of
Octopus Publishing Group Ltd
Carmelite House
50 Victoria Embankment
London EC4Y 0DZ
www.octopusbooks.co.uk

The authorized representative in the EEA is
Hachette Ireland, 8 Castlecourt Centre, Dublin
15, D15 XTP3, Ireland (email: info@hbgi.ie)

This edition published in 2025

This material was previously published as
Burnout's A Bitch

Distributed in the US by
Hachette Book Group
1290 Avenue of the Americas
4th and 5th Floors
New York, NY 10104

Distributed in Canada by
Canadian Manda Group
664 Annette St.
Toronto, Ontario, Canada M6S 2C8

ISBN 978-0-600-63958-9
eISBN 978-0-600-63959-6

A CIP catalogue record for this book is
available from the British Library.

Printed and bound in China

10 9 8 7 6 5 4 3 2 1

Editorial Director: Eleanor Maxfield
Senior Commissioning Editor: Louise McKeever
Editor: Ella Parsons
Art Director: Juliette Norsworthy
Designer: Lizzie B Design
Photographer: Andrew Hayes-Watkins
Food Stylist: Ellie Mulligan
Prop Stylist: Jennifer Haslam
Production Manager: Lisa Pinnell

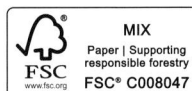

FSC
www.fsc.org
MIX
Paper | Supporting
responsible forestry
FSC® C008047

CONTENTS

Introduction

In a world where adversity and stress seem never ending, this book is your ultimate guide to resetting your energy, managing stress and navigating your mental health. It addresses the unexpected reasons you're tired all the time and identifies how to get back on track by making simple changes to your diet, lifestyle and mindset so that you can feel energized and mentally resilient every day.

I wrote this book because we are not only living in a burnout epidemic, but a mental health epidemic. Now more than ever before we are in need of change. The world can be an extremely overwhelming place. Living in a mental health crisis is not easy. Everyone is struggling. And the statistics are no joke:

- The World Health Organisation reports that around the world over 1 billion people are suffering from a mental health disorder, and in the first year of the Covid pandemic depression and anxiety increased by 25%.

- And in England, according to the charity Mind, 1 in 6 people report experiencing a common mental health problem (like anxiety and depression) in any given week. 1 in 5 people will experience suicidal thoughts and 1 in 15 attempt suicide.

Not to mention that burnout is now so common that the average professional burns out by the age of 32. PLUS stress can both cause and exacerbate a host of illnesses.

Which is why I felt obligated to give you, dear reader, all the tools you need to feel energized and mentally strong so you can cope during difficult times and not burnout like I did.

I want this book to be your toolkit for resetting your energy and falling in love with the life you have. Inside you will find:

- What is burnout and how to identify if you have it

- The reasons why you are tired all the time

- Which foods give you energy and which foods sap your energy

- Supplements to take for increased energy

- Simple tips to reduce stress, sleep better and manage your hectic life

- Practical steps for mastering your mindset

- A six-week meal plan complete with brand-new recipes to give you energy

- Weekly action points to help you live an energized and fulfilled life

I've poured my heart and soul into these pages. My hope is that you use this book as your energy and resilience bible. It's packed with practical wellness advice that you can extract and add to your own health toolkit.

Rosie

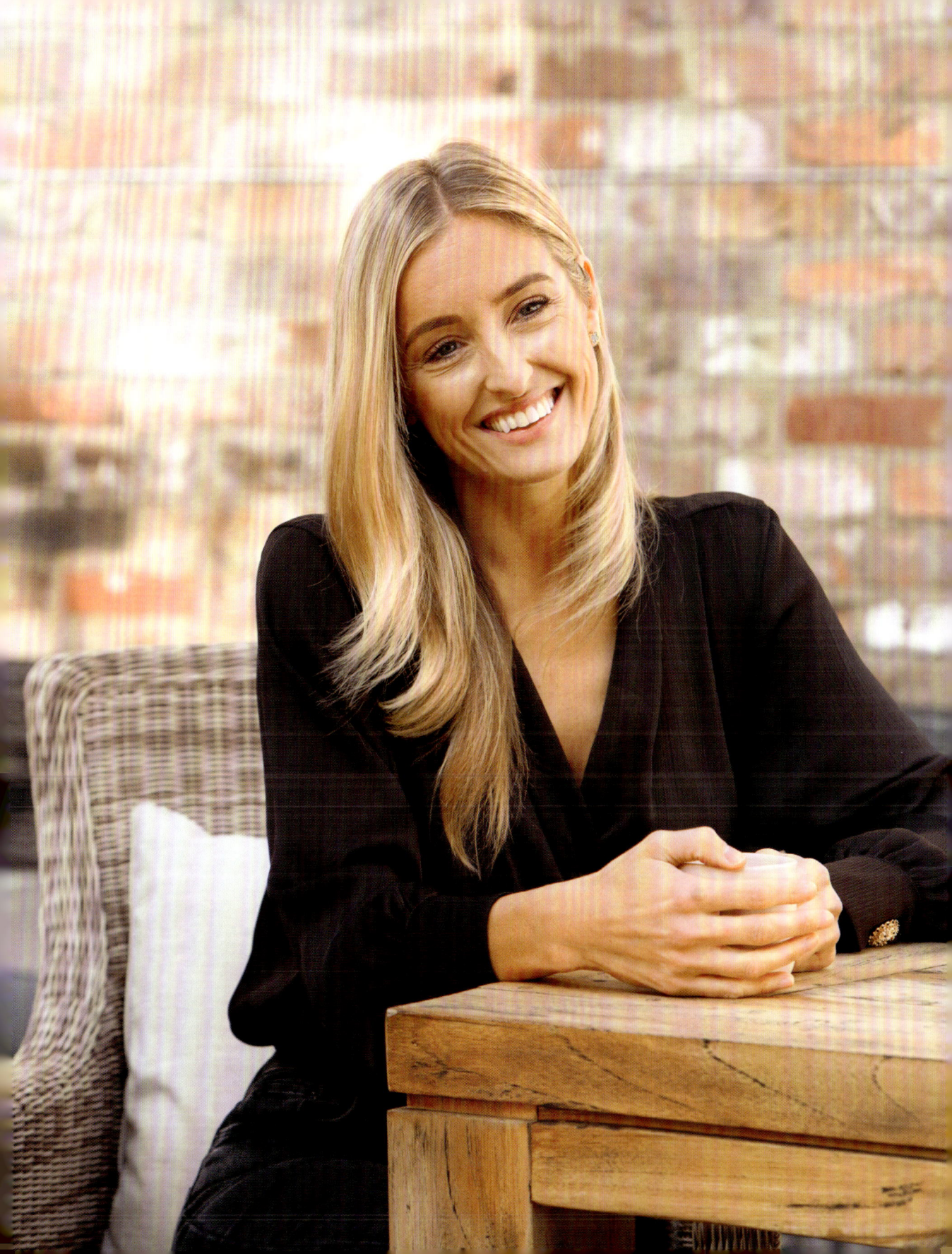

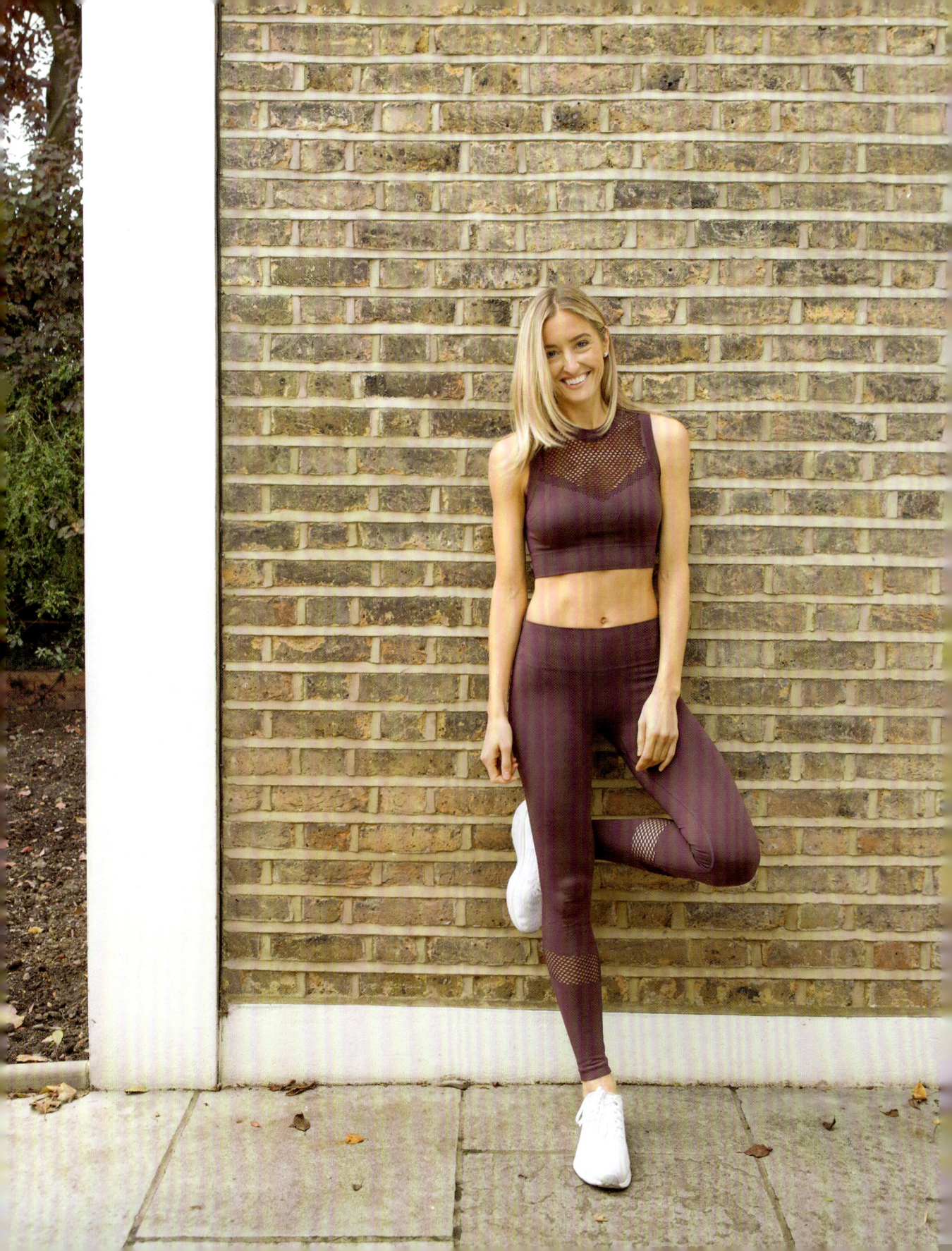

Using this Book

Who is this Book For?

This book is for anyone on the brink of giving up, and who can't see the light anymore. If you used to have energy and now feel disengaged, lonely and disconnected then this book is for you.

I wrote this book for individuals who lack energy and struggle with their mental health – maybe you've lost your drive, purpose, or motivation. This is for you if are stuck in a fatigue rut and can't seem to break out of the tireless rat race of external and internal demands.

It's for you if you struggle daily with anxiety, or suffer from a low mood or perpetual mood swings. And it's also for you if you are confused about which foods to eat and why, or feel misinformed about which supplements are best for you.

This book is also for anyone who has social media fatigue, or is fed up with their own negative self-talk. Are you ready to break free of toxic thought patterns, and adopt a healthy inner dialogue with yourself?

The Energy Reset Plan is for everyone who struggles with self-doubt and is in need of practical wellness advice to feel mentally resilient again.

How Long Will it Take to Recover?

The recovery time is different for everyone. For some people it can take years, others will see a difference in their energy levels in as little as a month. The answer really lies in the depth of your burnout. This book will kickstart you towards your recovery. By following all the advice, action points and tips in the book and completing the six-week meal plan, I expect each and every one of you to feel significantly more energized by the end of it.

This book is your survival guide for the overworked, overstimulated modern life we live. It's a tried-and-tested lifestyle plan to help you feel fabulous again. It's different to any other book because it helps you to identify WHY you are tired all the time and contains actionable strategies to get you back on your feet again. With my practical programme and powerful story of recovery, this book is here to inspire you and give you hope that you can recover too.

How to Use this Book

My advice is to read this book from beginning to end before you even start. It will be much more effective if you read all the theory text first. You can then work through the lifestyle action points and the to-do lists alongside the six-week meal plan.

Of course, in the future I'm happy for you to dip in and out through the chapters, but I want you to understand the reasoning before you apply all the strategies and this will ensure a complete food and lifestyle reset. Good luck!

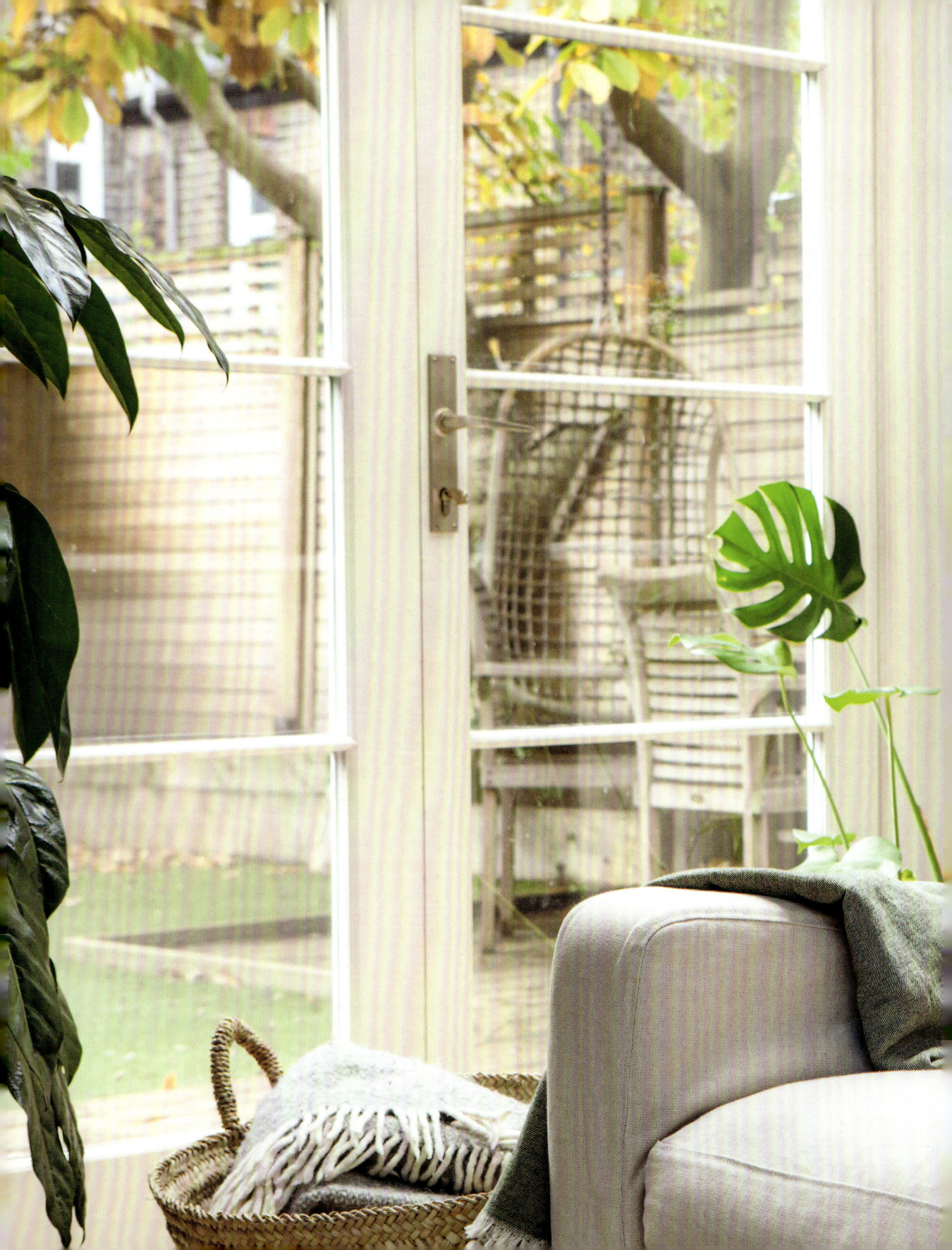

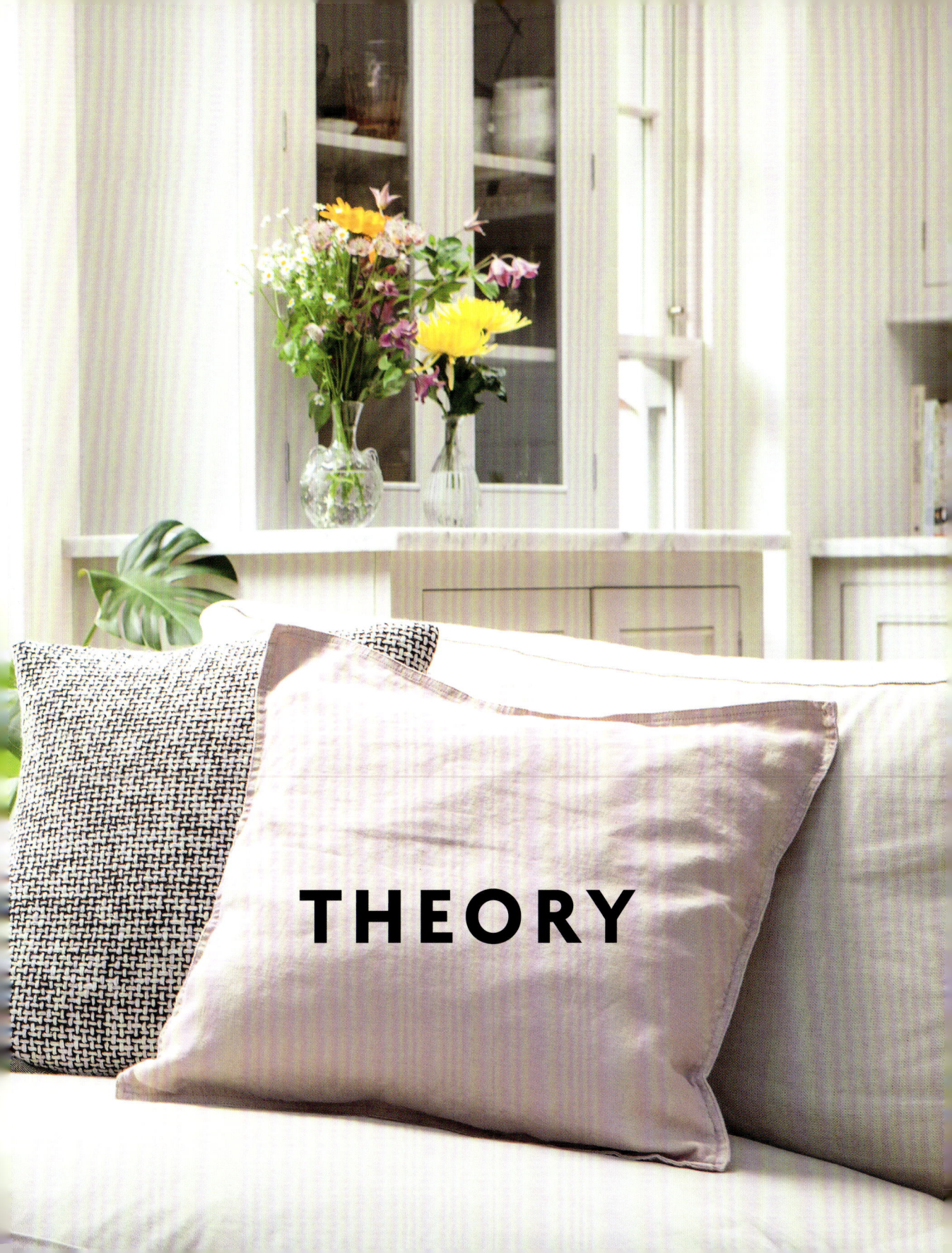

THEORY

Chapter One

My Story
& Road
to Recovery

'I had reached complete burnout'

March 6, 2014. I remember it like it was yesterday. I was walking in Hyde Park in London with a friend on a sunny but cold spring morning when all of a sudden I felt really dizzy. I turned to my friend and asked them if they also felt dizzy to check that it wasn't just me, but before I knew it my knees went from underneath me and I collapsed to the ground. Lying on the floor in a public place, unable to get up unaided, was not only mortally embarrassing but incredibly nerve-wracking. Nothing like that had ever happened to me before. I called a taxi to take me home, where I climbed into bed, hoping a good night's sleep would make me feel normal again. But it didn't. I basically stayed in bed for three years straight.

I slept and slept but no amount of sleep would make me feel better. I was completely paralyzed with exhaustion. I couldn't do anything. Even small tasks were challenging. Brushing my teeth was a huge effort. Going to the loo was an exhausting task. At my worst I was lying in bed struggling to lift my head off the pillow for a glass of water. What's more, my social life went out the window, I couldn't exercise – heck, I could barely even shower! My body couldn't move but my mind was in overdrive, full of thoughts such as 'What the hell is wrong with me?', 'How come I've been in bed for so long and still don't feel any better?' and 'How much longer am I going to be like this?'

I finally dragged myself to the doctor. When I sat in the consulting chair I remember barely being able to speak because I was so exhausted. I asked the doctor to run some blood tests on me and she agreed. I floated home hoping I'd get some answers. One week later when the results came back they were completely 'normal'. The doctor told me there was nothing physically wrong with me and suggested I was depressed. She prescribed me with antidepressants. I burst into tears at this miserable diagnosis and wailed 'But I'm not depressed, I'm EXHAUSTED!' I walked home, feeling helpless and alone and collapsed into bed again.

Days went by, then weeks, then months and I still wasn't feeling any better. I was so exhausted that even turning in my bed took a lot of mental and physical strength. I had never known such fatigue. When I realized that the exhaustion was here to stay it really affected my mental wellbeing. Lying in bed day after day, all alone, I was in a really dark place. With only my mind to entertain me, I often howled out in despair, crying at how miserable I was and how much suffering I felt. I remember constantly comparing my life to others on Instagram who had it all going for them, while I was trapped in bed like a waste of space. Eventually my thoughts turned so dark that I didn't want to be alive any more. But the thought of leaving this world just because I didn't have any energy was too unbearable to consider.

As I lay there, the frustration started to build inside. I could feel the anger in my blood. Screw that! I thought. I wasn't depressed. I knew something was wrong and I had to get to the bottom of it. Desperate to feel better, and with my doctor unable to offer an answer, I did what most people would do in that situation: I started to look for answers myself. So I got out my laptop, dug out all my nutrition books from school, did a ton of reading and decided to run some tests on myself.

I did a series of saliva tests to measure levels of the stress hormone cortisol, I did the Ragland's blood pressure test, I went to see a reflexologist and I consulted a naturopathic doctor.

Finally I ran one more test, just to be absolutely sure: the hair mineral analysis test. This one measures nutrient deficiencies in your body as well as heavy metal toxicity. I was really glad I did this test because the readings painted a picture of someone who had been burning the candle at both ends. My sodium and potassium levels were extremely low and I had high levels of mercury in my tissues. These findings are very common in people with a history of too much stress.

My findings all pointed to the same thing – I had reached complete burnout.

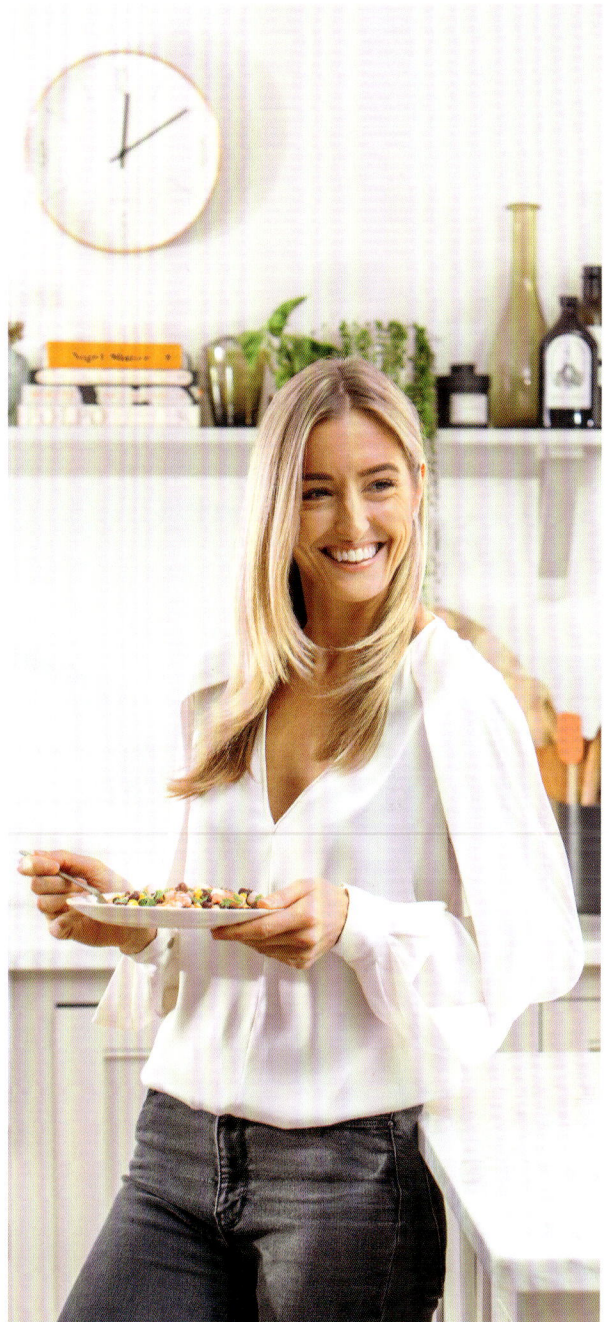

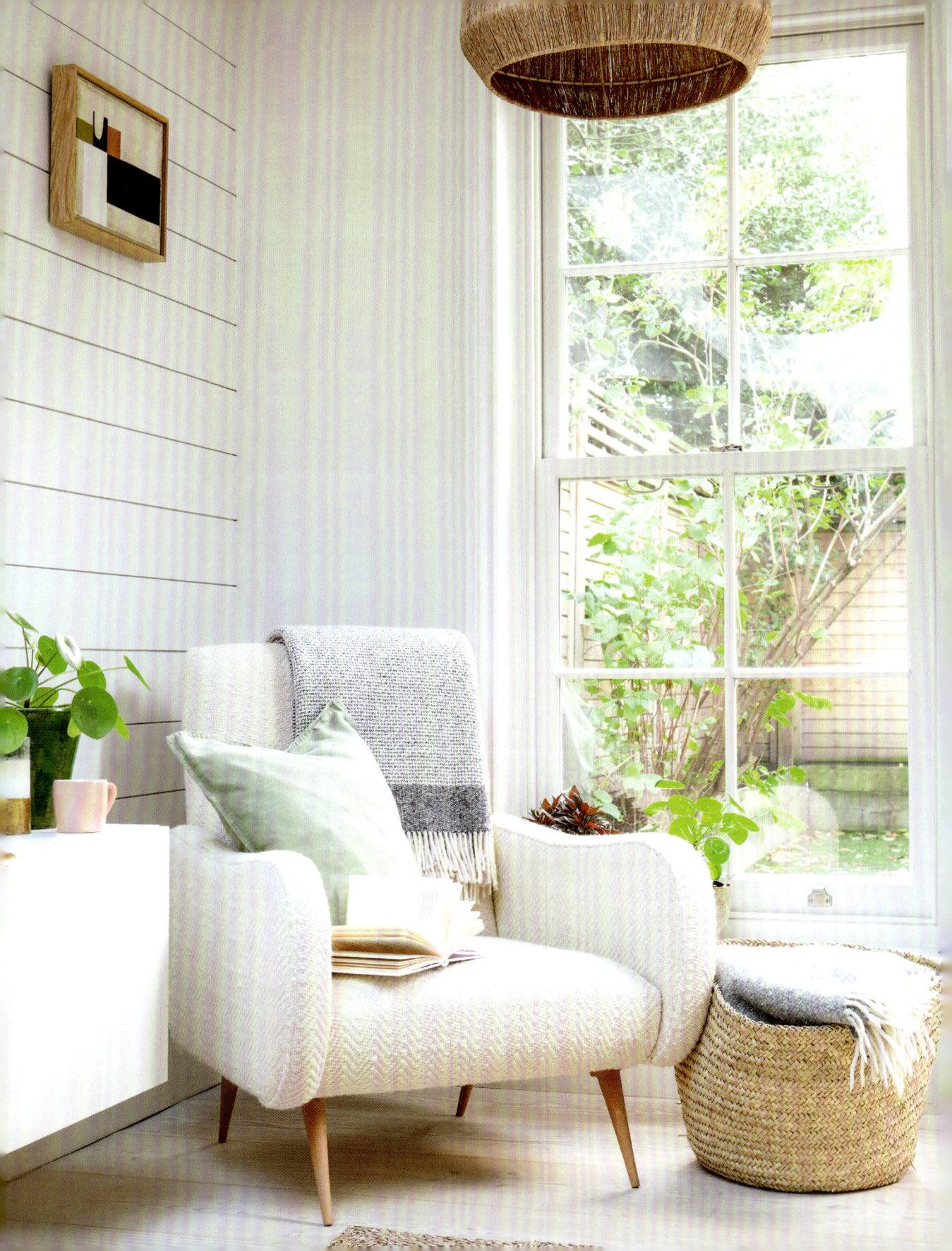

What is Burnout?

Put simply, burnout is when you experience significant amounts of stress over a long period of time, and you do not wind down and recover from those stressors. This puts a huge burden on your body (see page 27). If more stress is added to the equation then eventually you will end up exhausted.

It's a very frustrating condition because on the outside you look completely normal but on the inside you're completely debilitated. People think you are fine because you don't look ill. Often those who are burned out used to have a lot of energy but eventually feel like a shadow of their former selves because they are unable to do the simple things they used to.

But burnout doesn't just happen overnight; it's the culmination of years of running yourself ragged. One day, it creeps up on you and bites you in the ass! I have to admit I missed ALL of the warning signs: waking up after a good night's sleep but still feeling tired, dragging myself through the day, having huge energy slumps in the afternoon, feeling dizzy, being exhausted after exercise, not sleeping well, losing weight, having grey skin and dark circles under my eyes, and also having absolutely no drive or motivation to finish even small tasks. I was also undereating and overexercising, albeit unintentionally, both of which really don't help (more on this in later chapters).

'Burnout is the culmination of years of running yourself ragged'

How it Started for Me

Before I collapsed, my life was pretty good. I had soooo much energy. I set up my business Miss Nutritionist in 2010 and I started seeing clients on the day I got my certificate. My business started to go from strength to strength but it certainly wasn't easy. After graduating, I realized that I knew nothing about running a business and had to learn fast, so I hired a coach for the first six months. Having these coaching sessions changed how I approached things and made me really focus on what I wanted to achieve.

As the years went on I continued to see loads of clients one on one, put on my own talks and began working with large corporate companies. During this time I also developed my first line of food products, a range of protein bars created completely by accident. I invented them at home one day and started to sample them on my clients, who told me they were so good that I had to get them in the shops. So I found a factory, got some investment and launched them the same year. They started to sell extremely well.

Now that I was running two businesses there was a lot more pressure and I was being pulled in two directions. The workload was intense so I had little sleep and my diet went out of the window. At the same time I had some personal relationship problems. My fiancé at the time moved to a different country for his work which put a huge strain on us. I was meant to move with him but really didn't want to leave what I had built up, so our relationship started to fall apart. Eventually, I decided to end things in order to live a happier life, but the actual break up was so much more draining than I had expected.

To add to the stress, at the same time I also got thrown out of my house and had to move into temporary accommodation, which put a huge strain on my finances. So I said yes to every work opportunity going and literally didn't sleep because I felt such a huge sense of responsibility to keep everything together, and had a constant fear of bankruptcy. On top of that, I reached for unhealthy snacks the whole time to give me instant energy – and because, well, they just taste so damn good – even though I knew they were damaging my health in the long term.

Ignoring everything and working at the speed of light with no rest or good food, my body finally gave in and eventually I collapsed.

Are you surprised? Probably not. But I really was. When I set up Miss Nutritionist I was so enthusiastic about growing it into something mega that I poured my heart and soul into it. My entire existence evolved around my businesses because I was so passionate about improving other people's health through nutrition. Anyone on the outside would say I was working like a freight train. I said yes to everything, exercised like a machine, took on more than most, didn't sleep enough and ate a very unhealthy diet. I was living off chocolate and green tea, even though I was a nutritionist.

Physical vs Emotional Stress

After my collapse, one thing I learned is that there are different types of stress and your body cannot differentiate between them. Emotional stress can have a much greater impact on your adrenal glands than physical stress (see page 27). Nuts, right? That means than even if you are just worrying about something that'll probably never happen, your adrenal glands treat it in the same way as if you are constantly under physical attack.

Now knowing this, I believe one of the biggest contributors to my burnout was the emotional stress I endured from the breakdown of my ten-year relationship. It had been extremely challenging and the breakup punched a huge dent in me emotionally. It wasn't just the stress from working too hard that caused my burnout. For me, I burned out because I was experiencing multiple stressors over a long period of time.

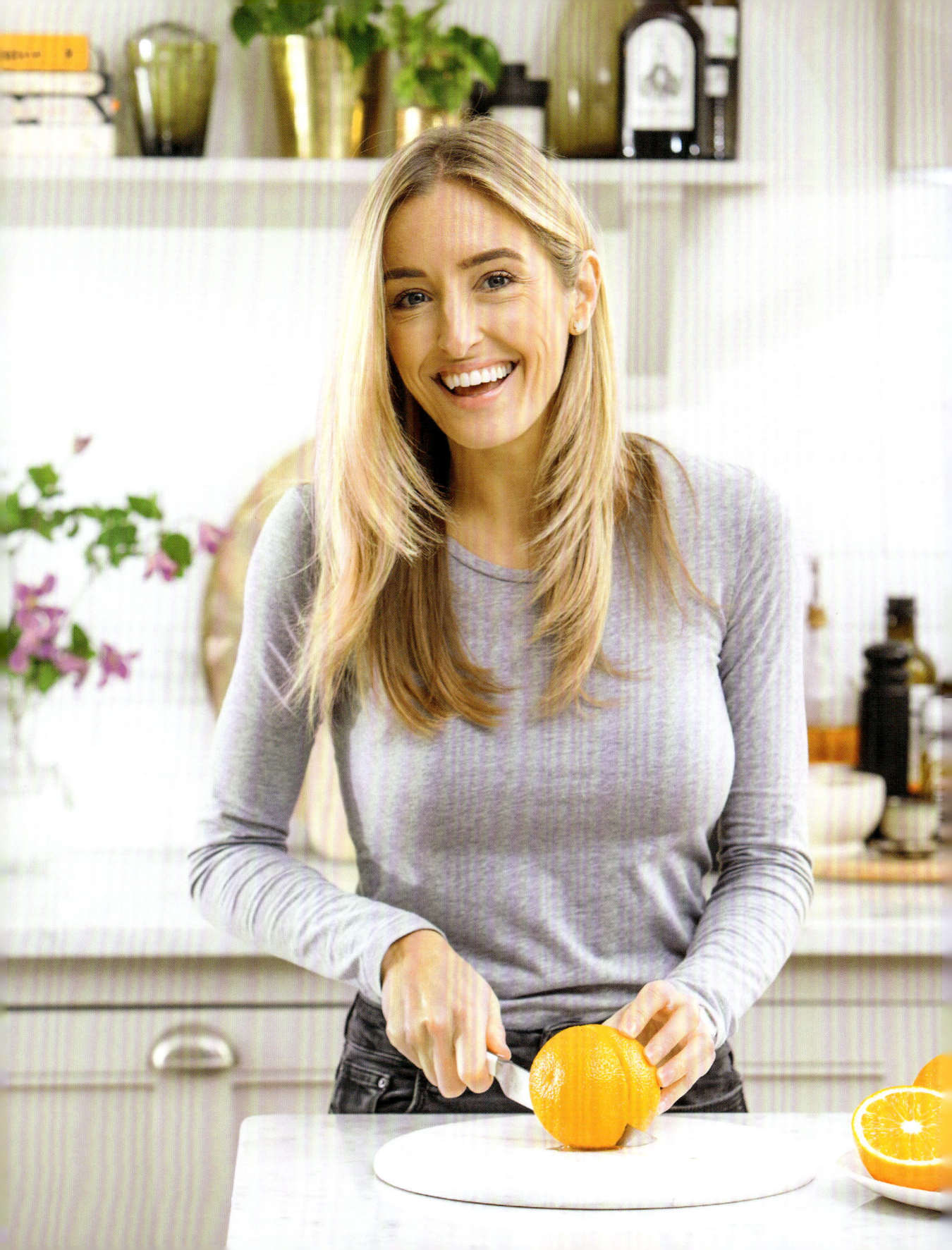

How I Got Back on My Feet

During my first year in bed I really had to slow down. Since I was so exhausted, I had no choice but to rest and sleep. I had to start saying no to things and learn to prioritize. And even though I was still running my businesses from my bed, my productivity was massively reduced. Each morning, I asked myself what the most important things were that day, and I'd only allow myself to do a maximum of three. Anything more was too taxing and too ambitious.

My work hours were reduced to about four per day. Almost every day I had to sleep during the afternoon and there were a lot of days when I was in bed all day and just couldn't move. This would usually be accompanied by lots of tears and feelings of helplessness.

If I started to get too tired, I would stop and just say to myself, 'I don't have to reply to this email now. I will do it in the morning when I wake up feeling better.' I had the help of a few interns at the time, whom I relied upon. They were my arms and legs if anything physical had to be done. Delegating was king. I did manage to go to meetings from time to time – probably too many – but I would always go straight home afterwards, collapsing in a taxi then getting straight into bed again, sometimes with my coat and shoes still on because I had nothing left in me to take them off. When I had to give nutrition consultations I asked clients to come to me, and even then it sapped all of my energy. I would always have to sleep afterwards and the rest of the day was a write off.

During that first year I felt totally alone. I started a new relationship that became emotionally draining, and my twin sister had just moved to the other side of the world for three years. I didn't tell my parents or the rest of my family because I didn't want to burden them, and I felt there was nothing they could do anyway. I lost a lot of friends because they didn't understand what was happening. They got fed up with me cancelling on them all the time and I eventually had no social life. It was an extremely lonely place.

As the years went on I relied on my twin sister for emotional support. Even though she lived miles away, I called her on a daily basis to tell her how I was doing. It was literally the only support around me. She was my lifeline, reassuring me I would recover while at the same time encouraging me to slow down and take things easy. As my illness went on for three years she ended up moving back to the UK to move in with me and look after me. If she hadn't been there for me physically and mentally I'm really not sure what would have happened. I was a total mess.

Over the course of the next three years I had to change everything about my life. I overhauled my diet, lifestyle, work schedule and social habits. I began with diet, as that was the easiest place to start. I had to eat more and consume food around the clock. If I didn't eat every three hours I would crash hard and have to go to bed, as sleep was the only thing that would reset my body. I was also taking nutritional supplements every day to help my body deal with stress: B vitamins, sodium, potassium, vitamin C, magnesium and so on. At one point I was taking 40 pills a day. This might sound a lot but I did notice a massive difference in my energy levels, so for me it was necessary.

The second thing I had to do was change my lifestyle. I really had to slow down and pull on the reins. I had to reduce my working hours, stop all exercise, cancel my social events and sleep a lot. My new motto was eat, sleep, rest, repeat. There was naturally a lot of resistance to this since my previous philosophy was work, work and work some more. I found this part extremely difficult to get my head around.

I also changed my sleeping patterns. Pre-burnout I would go to bed each night at midnight or later, and would have very broken or interrupted sleep. Today I'm extremely scrupulous about my sleep and have much more of a strict routine. I make sure I'm in bed by 10.30pm, put my phone on flight mode and aim to be asleep before 11pm. I keep the room dark, quiet and cool. This allows me to get a full eight hours a night. Even to this day I find that the quality of my sleep really determines how energized I feel the next day.

Lastly, I had to change my mindset. I found this aspect the hardest of all the changes. Our inner voices can be very loud and mine was often negative. I would constantly tell myself that I would never recover and that despite my efforts I would never be energized again. And the more I thought like this the more it sabotaged my recovery. Meditation really played a positive role for me. I called it my 'green time'. These were allocated times throughout the day when I would stop what I was doing and take 10 minutes to meditate or breathe deeply to get my body and mind into a more restful state (see page 88).

It was these three areas – diet, lifestyle and mindset – that had to change before I could say 'So long!' to burnout and 'Hello!' to the new, energized me. But it was a tough journey. Nothing is as hard as having to reinvent everything you know about yourself. There were so many dark nights of the soul and I really did reach rock bottom. I felt like a complete failure as, after all, I'd been working in the health and wellbeing sector. So how come I'd become so sick? Why had this happened to me?

Thankfully, today I'm 100 per cent recovered. But it's been the hardest journey of my life and extremely emotional. However, all the research, trial and error, therapies, medical visits, creams, pills and treatments have resulted in this book, which is basically my bible for recovering from burnout. I hope it will help you on your own road to recovery and keep you staying sane and positive along the way.

Nobody should have to endure what I did, yet modern life so often leads people down that path. But I'm here to say there is a way out. I've personally coached thousands of men and women to increase their energy, helped multiple companies improve the health of their staff, and written hundreds of blog posts on how to recover from burnout. It's my obligation to help as many people as possible to get their energy and lives back, and what better way than writing this book?

It also inspired me to create Go Mental – the UK's first mental wellbeing festival. Go Mental is an educational festival that brings together experts from various fields to teach you how to make your mental wellbeing journey easier.

I believe that our health system is broken. We are living in a mental health epidemic and normal, conventional medicine isn't working. I'm determined to solve this mental health crisis we are living in.

Go Mental is a full day packed with inspirational talks, Q&A panels, interactive workshops and fitness and meditation classes. I want people to be able to extract all the information they need to feel mentally well.

It also introduces you to the best brands and products on the market that are going to change your mental wellness game. AND it's about community! Everyone who attends Go Mental wants to be a part of something, and feel connected to this mental health movement.

If you would like to join us at Go Mental this year check out www.go-mental.co.uk

'I hope this book will help you on your own road to recovery, and keep you positive along the way'

Chapter Two

What is Burnout?

'You get burnout when your plate is already full but you keep adding to it'

Today, more than ever before, we live in an age where everything is nonstop. From the minute we wake up in the morning to the moment we go to sleep at night, we are bombarded left, right and centre by multiple stimuli. Be they work demands, relationships, children, to-do lists or social media, all these stimuli can be thought of as 'micropressures'.

When all of these add up, it's almost impossible to switch off. This is where the danger lies. And as a result, more and more people are suffering from burnout and other stress-related conditions. We need to get a grip on how to prevent burnout and how to keep ourselves energized all day, every day.

Name one person you know who isn't stressed or tired. We are living in a burnout epidemic.

Burnout is on the Rise

- In 2019 the World Health Organization included burnout in its International Classification of Diseases for the first time.

- In 2022 burnout was reported by 40% of workers globally[1]

- In 2023 61% of working people in Britain reported feeling exhausted at the end of the working day.[2]

- In 2024, 1 in five workers in the UK needed to take time off due to poor mental health.[3]

(1) Future Forum Pulse Survey, October 2022
(2) Trades Union Congress Report, 2023
(3) The Mental Health UK Annual Report, 2024

Why are we so tired and stressed?

Burnout is the inability to cope with the pressures of modern life and is predominantly caused by the build-up of a multitude of factors that the body deems as stressful.

Burnout is a stress-related condition. But before we talk about the downside of stress, it's important to remember that acute stress is actually a good thing. It's a defence mechanism to protect us from the dangers of the world. It's totally normal and actually healthy for your body to undergo a stress response from time to time. It's when stressors build up and linger for a long time that problems occur.

The Science of Stress

Stress starts in the brain. Every 3–6 seconds, an area in the brain called the hypothalamus checks for danger. When it detects a stressful situation (a sabre-tooth tiger approaching, for example) the hypothalamus will release corticotropin-releasing hormone (CRH). This hormone sends a message to the nearby pituitary gland to produce another hormone called adrenocorticotropic hormone (ACTH). ACTH is then detected by the adrenal glands.

The adrenal glands are endocrine glands which sit on top of the kidneys. There are two adrenal glands, both about the size of a walnut, which are chiefly responsible for regulating the stress response through the synthesis of numerous hormones. The adrenal glands secrete two main hormones into the bloodstream: adrenaline and cortisol. These hormones prepare us for the stress response. The heart beats faster, our pupils dilate and glucose is sent directly to the muscles so we have the physical energy to mount a 'fight or flight' response, allowing us to better fight off the tiger, or run away quicker.

When the threat disappears, levels of both cortisol and adrenaline start to lower and instead another hormone called dehydroepiandrosterone (DHEA) is released from the adrenal glands to moderate the stress response. Amazing isn't it? Our bodies are sending messages all the time, just like texting, in order to communicate and deliver information.

This carefully orchestrated sequence of hormonal messages happens in a nano second and is critical for us to either fight or flee from danger. BUT our bodies can't differentiate between physical danger and emotional stressors, so we mount a stress reaction in the same way when we miss our train or have an argument with our boss. The constant stressors we encounter every day can put strain on our bodies, resulting in a wide range of serious health problems, including burnout.

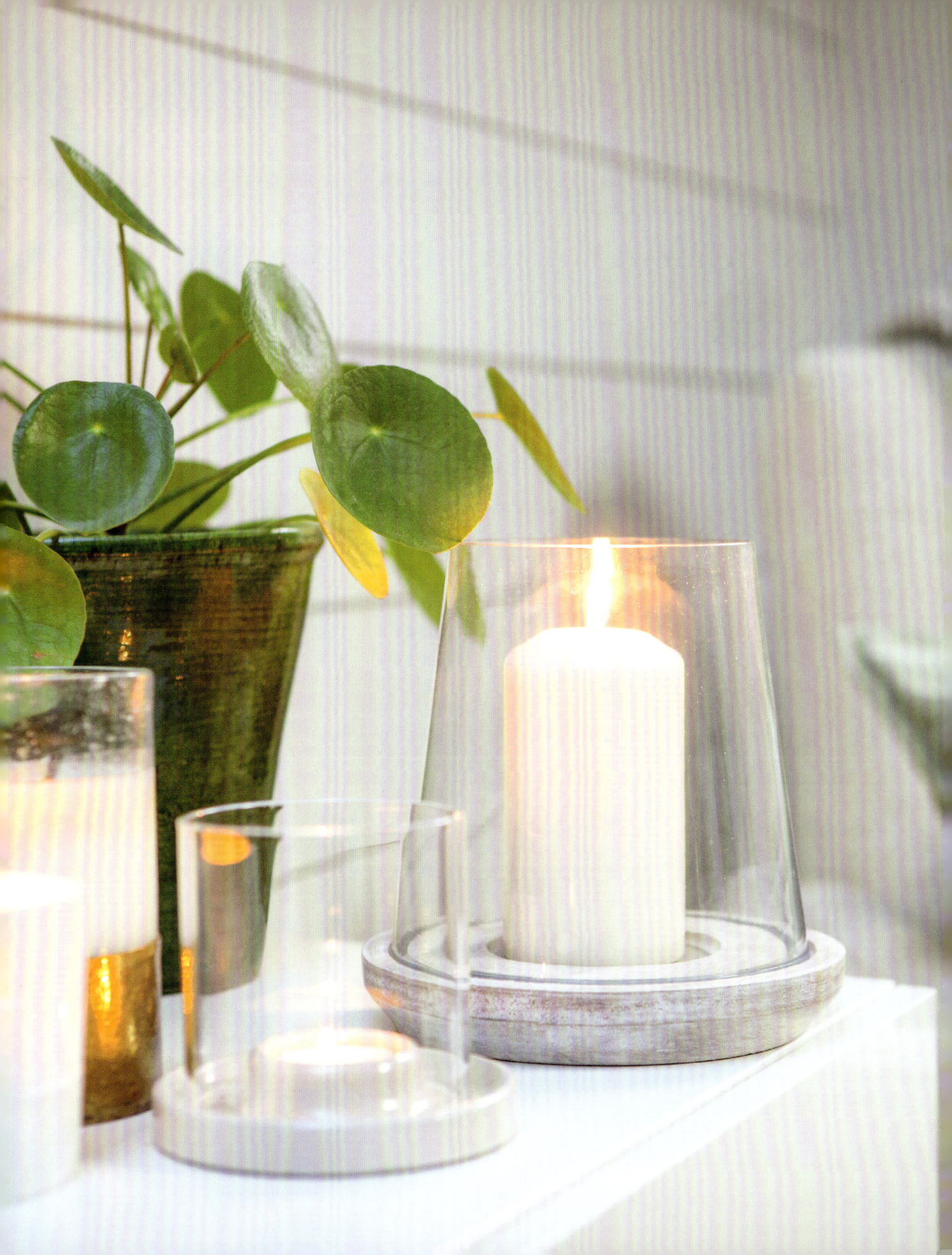

How Do You Recognize Burnout?

When you have burnout, you really know about it. You used to have energy but now you're a shadow of your former self. You're dragging yourself through each day with no energy or enthusiasm to do anything... that's my most honest description.

The most common symptoms of burnout are:

- You're extremely exhausted all the time
- You still feel tired even after a good night's sleep
- You experience dizzy spells quite often
- You drag yourself through each day
- You lose your drive and motivation
- Even small tasks are challenging
- Your cognitive function and memory start to fail you
- You experience severe energy slumps and crashes on a daily basis
- You have lower back pain
- You feel completely exhausted after exercise

WHO Definition of Burnout

The World Health Organization defines burnout as 'a syndrome conceptualized as resulting from chronic workplace stress that has not been successfully managed. It is characterized by three dimensions:

- feelings of energy depletion or exhaustion
- increased mental distance from one's job, or feelings of negativism or cynicism related to one's job
- reduced professional efficacy.'

Why is it Important to Recognize the Signs?

The answer is simple: because burnout literally stops you from living a normal life. The exhaustion is so extreme you can't do simple tasks like having a shower, going out to meet friends or exercising. All the things you used to take for granted become very challenging.

It's also important because more and more people are suffering from this condition, yet not much is known about it. In fact, according to the Health and Safety Executive (HSE), 602,000 workers in Great Britain suffered from work-related stress, depression or anxiety in 2018/19, and 12.8 million working days were lost over that period as a result.

However, the definition is still in its early stages. There is more research to be done, but there are some key things we do know and there are major changes that we, as individuals, can make to have a positive impact now. This book is a holistic approach to improving your lifestyle and habits to help you recover, or better protect yourself, from the effects of stress and exhaustion.

Ruling Out Other Medical Conditions

Burnout is hard to diagnose due to its similarities with so many other conditions. So how do you know if it's burnout or something else? First things first, it is critical that you visit your doctor to discuss how you are feeling and what symptoms you are experiencing. A blood test can be done to check for conditions such as anaemia, under-active thyroid, low vitamin D or B12 levels, a virus and so on – all of which can have similar symptoms to burnout.

Chronic fatigue syndrome (CFS), also known as ME, which stands for myalgic encephalomyelitis, is much more multifactorial than burnout. Patients might present with an array of underlying factors contributing to fatigue, such as immune dysregulation, inflammation, blood sugar issues, digestive issues and an underactive thyroid. So it's a much more complex picture. While there is a lot of crossover with the symptoms of burnout, patients with CFS or ME typically tend to experience muscle pain and migraines, while burnout individuals do not (but this is not definitive). Seeing a doctor will help determine if you are suffering from CFS.

TAKE ACTION
Even if you are convinced that you are suffering from burnout, and not any other condition, it is still important to seek medical advice in the first instance.

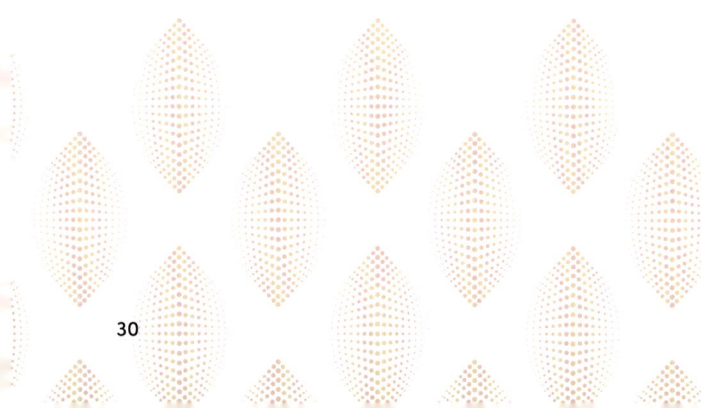

Different Types of Stressors

It's probably not news to you that there are different types of stressors. However, it's important to know that one person's stressor might not be stressful to another. It's all relative. So let's take a look at the different types of stressor so you can be aware of them going forward. All these things can trigger a stress response:

Physical These are real threat-based stressors such as incidents, accidents, trauma, injuries, overexertion, dehydration, wounds and so on.

Psychological A crisis of values, purpose, meaning or existence.

Physiological Headaches, dizziness, nausea, vomiting, constipation, tiredness, stiff or tense muscles.

Cognitive Anxious thoughts, fears, memory loss, information overload, poor concentration.

Emotional Loss of a loved one, arguments, feelings of tension, relationship difficulties, family disputes, friction between co-workers.

Behavioural Sleep problems, grinding teeth, substance abuse, smoking, addictions.

Social Feelings of being alone, lack of communication, feeling an outsider, lack of support, isolation, not feeling integrated or welcome.

Cellular Low blood sugar, toxins, pesticides, nutritional deficiencies.

Immunological Inflammation, allergies, food intolerances or viral, fungal or bacterial infections.

Environmental Air volume and quality, contaminants, pollution, radiation, severe weather alerts, natural disasters, war.

So you can see there are quite a lot of things that can cause us stress.

Next Steps
Using the examples above, I'd like you to think about the stressors that you were not aware of that might be affecting you. Write them down.

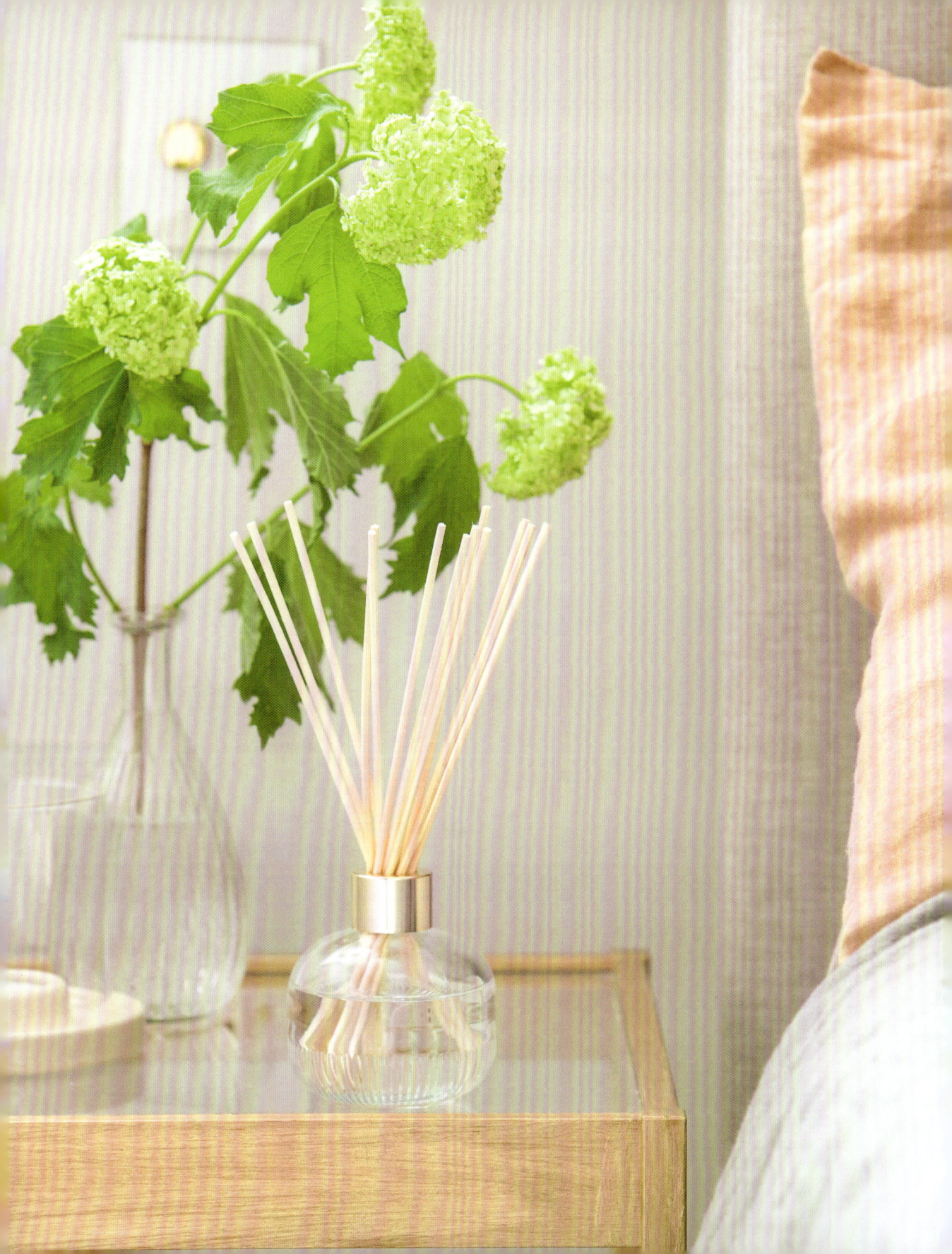

It's Different for Everyone

Everyone's stress is different. What stresses you out might not stress out another, but each stressor mounts the same stress response. For example, if you have an argument with someone and fall out it will cause the same adrenal response as if you were going for a long run in the park. It all adds up.

Most people don't realize they are stressed or, if they do feel stress, they don't take the time to stop and think about it. Identifying your stressors is key to reducing them.

Here is a list of 'micropressures' which can build up over time and contribute to your overall stress levels:

– Social media
– To-do lists
– Family demands
– Demanding travel schedules
– Dashing from meeting to meeting
– Arguments with loved ones
– Work deadlines
– Maintaining a certain reputation
– Building a business
– Children
– Household chores
– Admin
– Running errands

What we don't realize is that these micropressures, when added together, put us in a constant state of stress.

Can you Recover from Burnout?

Absolutely! You really can. But recovery is a multifactorial journey. There are a lot of things you have to change. How you change is how you succeed. Recovery all boils down to making changes to your diet, lifestyle and mindset. It's not easy and usually it's one step forward, two steps back. But as long as you eliminate or reduce your stressors, change your diet, manage your thoughts and set up a strong support network you will get there.

How Long will it Take?

Usually it takes about 2–3 years to develop burnout and about 2–3 years to recover from it. BUT everyone is different. Please remember that no amount of pushing will heal burnout – patience and persistence is the bottom line.

The Energy Barometer

Now it's time to identify where you're at. I want you to take the quiz below to reveal where you are on the energy barometer. Find out if you're just a little pooped or flat out on the floor. Give yourself one point for all the questions you answer yes to.

Questions:

1. Do you wake up, even after a good night's sleep, and still feel tired? ☐
2. Do you find small tasks challenging? ☐
3. Does it take you much longer to complete tasks than it used to? ☐
4. Do even simple things completely wipe you out? ☐
5. Do you experience dizzy spells during the day? ☐
6. Do you feel light-headed when you stand up too quickly? ☐
7. Do you feel tired all the time? ☐
8. Are you dragging yourself through the day? ☐
9. Do you rely heavily on stimulants such as tea, coffee and sugar to keep you going on a daily basis? ☐
10. Do you feel increasingly overwhelmed at work? ☐
11. Do you find small things upset you? ☐
12. Have you lost your drive and motivation? ☐
13. Do you feel like a zombie most days? ☐
14. Did you used to have a lot of energy and now feel like a shadow of your former self? ☐
15. Do you feel really fatigued after exercise? ☐
16. Are you ever so tired you can't even read a text message? ☐
17. Do you ever feel so tired you feel sick? ☐
18. Do you find yourself increasingly unhappy? ☐
19. Is your memory not as good as it used to be? ☐
20. Do you have brain fog and reduced cognitive function? ☐
21. Does it take you a few hours to actually wake up in the morning? ☐
22. Have you experienced significant amounts of stress over the past three years? ☐
23. Do you have low blood pressure? ☐
24. Do you feel like you have to force yourself to keep going? ☐
25. Do you have severe energy slumps if you skip meals? ☐
26. Do you cancel social events because you simply can't face the thought of them? ☐
27. Do you find yourself desperate for a nap during the day? ☐
28. Is your energy the lowest in the morning when you wake up? ☐

Total Score: _____

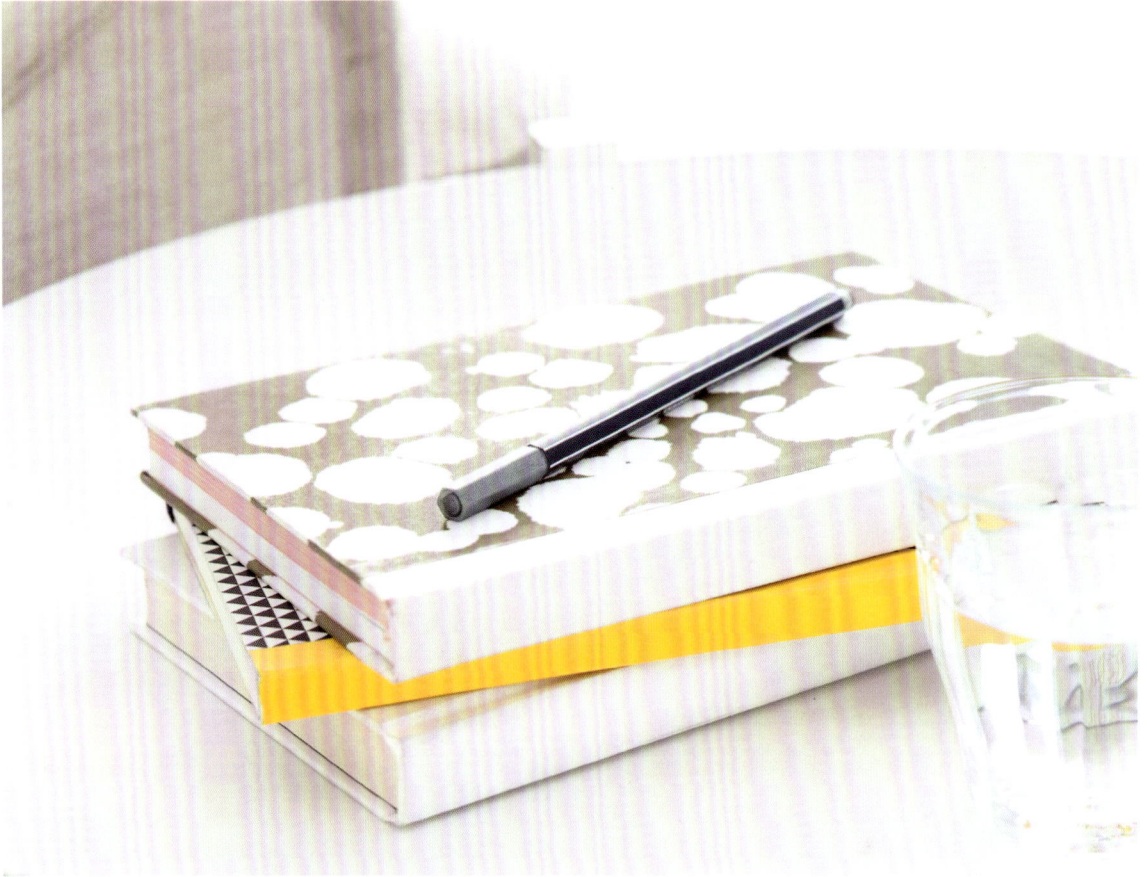

Scores

0-8 Healthy Stage

Your score is very low and indicates you have a healthy stress response. Well done! Your resilience is good and you are doing the right things to protect yourself against burnout. Stress itself is not the enemy. The danger lies with too much stress and an inability to cope.

9-18 Resistance Stage

Your score indicates that your body is having to go to large efforts to cope with the stressors in your life. You have mild burnout and will head towards complete exhaustion if you don't intervene now.

19-28 Exhaustion Stage

You're on the floor and need a complete overhaul. It's imperative that you make some significant changes to get out of this exhausted state that you're in. Luckily, all the advice in this book coupled with the meal plan will help you to get your energy back and get you back on your feet.

How to Reset Your Energy

Identify Your Stressors

First things first: identify your stressors. Everyone is different. Your neighbour will have completely different stressors to you. But I want you to take the time to identify what YOUR stressors are and what things are robbing YOUR energy. Because then we can think about how we either eliminate them or reduce them.

TAKE ACTION
Get a pen and write down the three things that cause you most stress in your life right now. Here are some examples:

– You hate your job
– You don't want to be in your existing relationship any more
– Your boss puts too much pressure on you
– You don't have a healthy relationship with a family member
– You are not making enough money to pay the bills
– You're desperate to find the partner of your dreams but don't believe they exist

It's important to know that your body does not differentiate between stressors. It can't tell the difference between having an argument with a loved one and running for a plane that's about to leave for your wedding.

Eliminate or Reduce Your Stressors

Now that you have identified your main stressors, there are two ways to get you feeling energized again.

1. Removing the stressors from your life, or
2. Reducing the amount of time you are exposed to those stressors.

TAKE ACTION
Ask yourself this question: Can I eliminate the number one stressor in my life completely?

If the answer is YES then my next question is: What do you need to do in order to move the needle on this? Do you need to change jobs? Get interviews? Talk to your friends and ask who's hiring? Update your CV or résumé? What is it that you actually need to do in order to remove this stressor from your life?

Please write down some ideas.

If you answered NO to this question and you simply cannot eliminate the main stressor in your life, I want you to think about how you can handle it differently. Can you reduce the amount of time you are exposed to that stressor?

If your main stressor is that you have a very toxic relationship with a parent or sibling, can you find a way to spend less time with them? For example, the next time you see them are you able to invite other family members too so that it dilutes your time with that person?

Or if they are constantly calling you or nagging you about something, can you tell them that you have so much on your plate right now that you are only able to take phone calls between the hours of 9am and 10am on a Friday morning?

I really want you to think outside the box here and establish what you can actually do – however small it seems – in order to help yourself. I want you to take action and not be the victim. I don't want your energy robber to keep on robbing you. It's time to make some changes so you can move forward in your recovery.

Deal with Stress

The good news is, managing your stressors – particularly the micropressures – may be simpler than you think. First, you have to understand that there are two ways to deal with stress:

1. React
2. Respond

Put your hand up if you know a 'stressy' person? Or perhaps that 'stressy' person is you! My point is, if you REACT to a stressful situation and perceive it as negative, it's an overreaction, meaning it will cause more of an adrenaline surge by mounting a stress response. However, if you choose to RESPOND to a stressful situation, then you are choosing to deal with it better and therefore it's less likely to mount that stress response in the body – which is what we want.

TAKE ACTION

The number one way to reduce stress is to put it into perspective. And to do that you can ask yourself these three questions:

– Is that stressor the end of the world? (NO)
– Will it change in time? (YES)
– Is there someone worse off than you? (YES)

Easy, right? And it really works. Instantly your stressor dissipates and the reaction is immediately reduced. Try it next time you feel like your world is going to end. This takes a little practice but is so effective. I want this to become the norm for you as soon as possible.

How Stress Affects Motivation

Cortisol is our motivation hormone. It's our 'get up and go' hormone. It's responsible for giving us drive in our lives.

There is a natural circadian rhythm for cortisol. Healthy cortisol levels should be highest in the morning – the cortisol gives your body a boost to help you get out of bed feeling great – and lowest at bedtime when you need to be resting.

Constant stress alters your body's natural circadian rhythm, which is the reason you feel exhausted in the morning yet wired but tired at night.

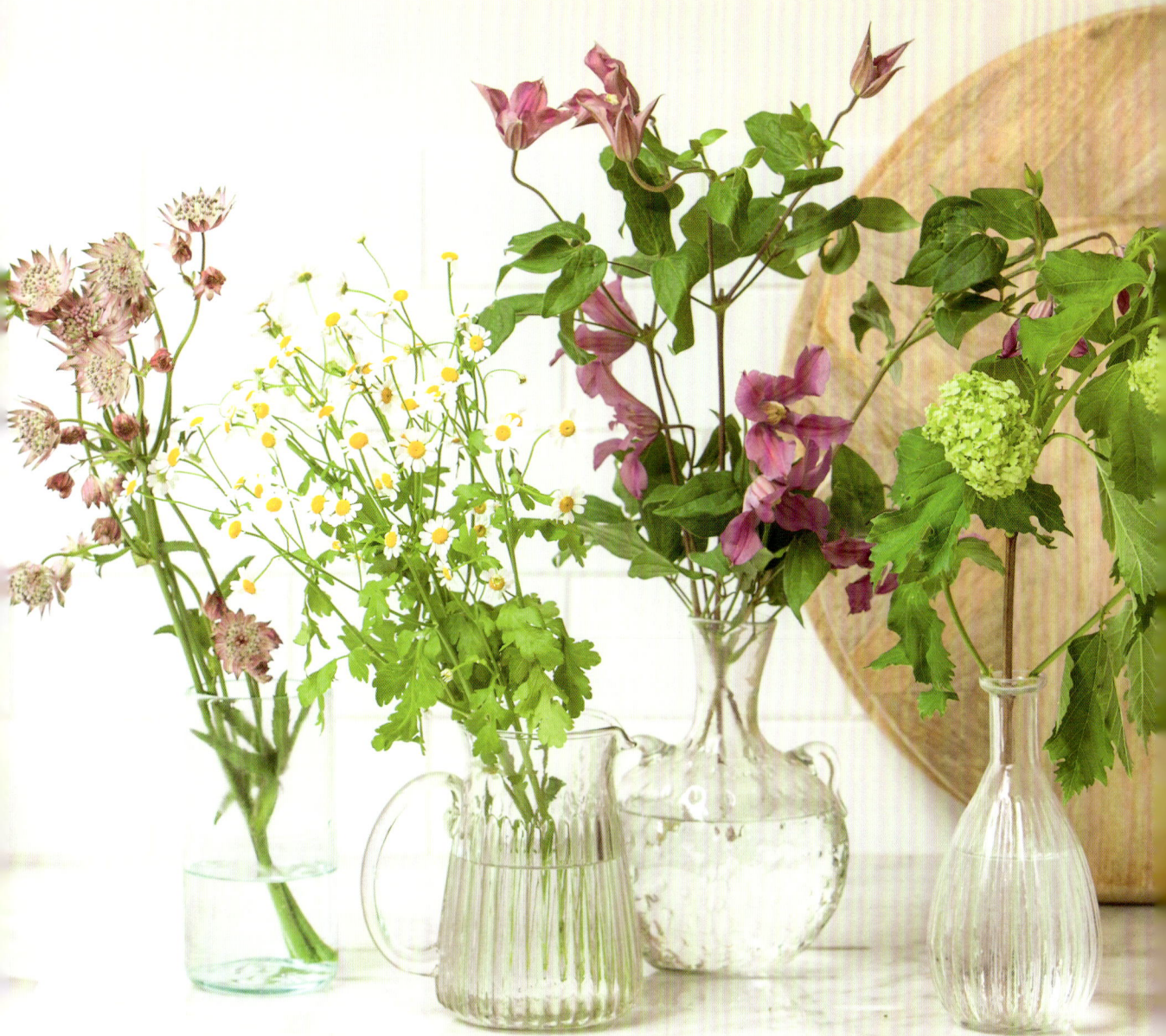

Get Your Motivation Back

If you are exhausted and feel like you've lost your drive and motivation as a result, here are some tips to get you thinking about your life and what you want.

TAKE ACTION
Use the below as helpful starting points:

1. Focus on your WHY. Why did you choose a career in the industry you're in? What is your purpose? What is it that you want to achieve? What actually gets you out of bed in the morning? Take some time out to identify what your why really is and write it down.

2. Hire a coach or find a mentor for a few sessions to help inspire you again. This always boosts my motivation and gets me to refocus. Get in touch with a coach and ask if you can have an preliminary chat to see if it's for you.

3. Chat it out. Talk to people about your passion and your goals and always surround yourself with positive and inspirational people on a daily basis to keep you going. You are who you surround yourself with.

4. Visualize your goal. The more specific you can be the better. The more details you can imagine and the more you visualize it, the stronger it will become. Never let go of this image in your mind.

5. Keep learning. What I mean by this is keep reading. Reading a personal development book, for example, will provide you with inspiration. You will continue to learn nuggets of information which will motivate you on a personal level.

To Do

1. Write down what you are going to do this week in order to feel motivated again. This week I am going to…

2. Write down the three main stressors in your life. Think about ways in which you can eliminate them or reduce them.

3. Highlight the stressors in your life using the list on page 31. Which ones were you unaware of before?

Chapter Three

Food for Energy

'Every meal is an opportunity to feed or fail your body'

The first pillar of burnout recovery is your diet. There are so many myths and misconceptions about healthy eating, so I'm here to give you a tour of the dos and don'ts of eating when it comes to restoring energy. You will learn what to eat and why, and how to put it all into practice with my six-week programme.

Blood Sugar

The number one way to achieve sustainable energy levels throughout the day is to balance our blood sugar levels.

Every time you eat, the sugars from the foods you have eaten are released into your bloodstream in the form of a simple sugar called glucose. This triggers the pancreas to release a hormone called insulin to transfer the glucose out of your blood and into the cells of your body where it is used for energy.

Your body can only deal with one to two teaspoons of glucose in the blood at any one time. However, the more sugary the foods you eat, the higher your blood sugar level will rise. If, for example, you drank a fizzy drink containing 21 teaspoons of sugar, the sugar level in your blood would rise steeply. The problem with rapidly rising sugar levels is that they will come down at an equal speed. The initial energy rush that the sugar gives you will be followed by an energy slump as large amounts of insulin are released, bringing the sugar levels crashing down.

This is when we start to experience the physical and mental symptoms of low blood sugar levels, including dizziness, faintness, headaches, nausea, blurred vision, sweating, palpitations, cravings and irritability. This happens about an hour after sugary foods have been eaten as these foods dump a large amount of glucose into the bloodstream all at once, triggering a strong insulin reaction which then lowers blood sugar levels rapidly.

During this energy slump, the usual response is to reach for more sweet foods or stimulants such as tea, coffee and chocolate to boost energy levels. However, this only raises blood sugar levels right up again and perpetuates the blood sugar rollercoaster.

Of course, symptoms of low blood sugar also occur when we skip meals as we are simply not eating enough to replenish our blood sugar level and provide our cells with the energy they need. Whatever you do, don't skip meals. When blood sugar levels drop, this will tell the adrenal glands to mount a stress response and release cortisol into the bloodstream. This is what we want to avoid.

How to Balance Blood Sugar

Balancing your blood sugar level is key to maintaining energy throughout the day. If you keep your blood sugar on an even keel you are likely to have better energy levels. Here are my top tips for balancing blood sugar:

1. Eat little and often around the clock – ideally every 3–4 hours. Try breakfast, snack, lunch, snack, dinner.

2. Eat protein at every meal and snack – especially breakfast. Chicken, eggs, lentils, tofu, nuts and fish are all good sources.

3. Swap refined carbohydrates such as white bread, pasta and cakes for complex carbohydrates such as lentils, chickpeas, brown rice and wholemeal pasta.

4. Eat at least 5–8 portions of fresh vegetables every day.

5. Reduce your intake of coffee and tea, drinking water instead during the day.

How Can you Tell if Your Blood Sugar Levels are Low?

It's quite simple. Do you...

> Get tired and irritable when you don't eat?

> Crave sugary sweet foods, coffee, chocolate and tea?

> Yawn a lot?

> Have an energy slump in the middle of the afternoon?

> Have regular mood swings?

> Struggle if you go too long without eating?

> Become less productive at work when you don't eat?

> Have poor concentration and memory?

> Drink tea or coffee or smoke during the day?

> Suffer from insomnia?

If the answers are 'yes', then your blood sugar levels are very likely to be low.

Foods that Sap Energy

There are certain foods that wreak havoc with your blood sugar levels, and therefore energy. Watch out for the following:

1. **Refined sugar.** Cut out sweets, fizzy drinks etc. The only sugars I want you to eat on this plan are fruits or a little bit of honey.

2. **Alcohol**. Wreaks havoc with blood sugar levels, robs vitamins and minerals from the body and causes inflammation. No thanks.

3. **Refined carbs.** Cakes, biscuits, doughnuts etc. See page 52 for more on gluten.

4. **Caffeine.** See page 50 for more detail

5. **Energy drinks.** Usually packed with sugar AND caffeine.

6. **Processed foods.** These have been stripped of nutrient content and likely contain artificial flavourings and chemicals.

Foods that Give Energy

There are three macronutrients which provide your body with the building blocks to recover and are all vital for energy. They are:

1. **Proteins.** Found in foods such as red meat, fish, chicken, eggs and protein smoothies, proteins provide us with essential amino acids – 'essential' because our bodies cannot make them (see page 56).

2. **Healthy fats.** Found in avocados, oily fish, nuts and seeds, healthy fats provide us with essential fatty acids.

3. **Slow-release carbohydrates.** These release their sugars into the bloodstream much more slowly than refined carbs because they contain fibre. This includes beans, quinoa, lentils and chickpeas.

Over the next six weeks I want your food to be as fresh and as nutrient-dense as possible. I like to stick to the following rule... If it didn't come from the ground or didn't have a mother, don't eat it!

What about Intermittent Fasting?

This is when you fast for a period of time each day, usually for about 16 hours, eating all your meals within the remaining 8-hour period.

Health benefits can include weight loss, as fasting helps cut calories and restrict food intake. The body also undergoes cellular repair during fasting, removing waste from cells and restoring them. For this reason, fasting may contribute to longevity. It also increases levels of a protein in the brain called BDNF, which is believed to improve memory and learning skills.

The bottom line is that Intermittent fasting can be effective and I use it in my clinic as a tool for weight loss over a short period of time. However, it's not easy and definitely not for everyone, especially those with energy deficiencies. You guys need more fuel so please park any thoughts on fasting for now. You can reintroduce it into your life again when you have recovered.

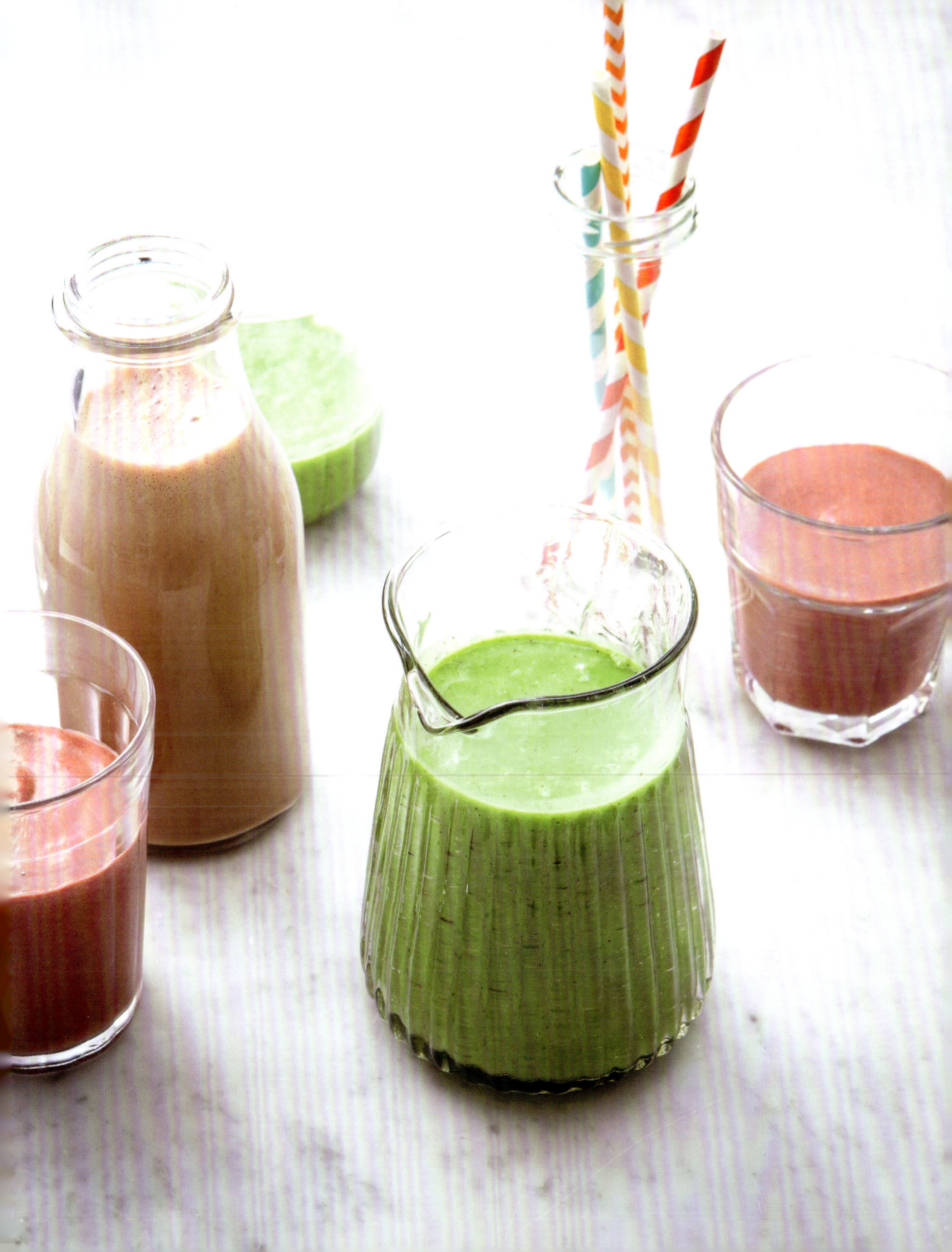

Nutrition and Mental Health

Food isn't just energy, it's information. It communicates messages to your genes, hormones, immune system, gut flora and every system in our body! What you eat dictates how you think, feel and behave. Making the right food choices can make you feel emotionally stronger and lift your esteem.

Foods to Reduce to Feel Better

Sugar Multiple studies have documented the link between high sugar diets and depression. Reducing sugar intake will also help balance insulin levels, helping with mood swings. The difficult thing about sugar is that it's highly addictive but weaning yourself off slowly can have a profound impact on your overall health.

TAKE ACTION Start slowly and swap artifically sugary foods for those with natural sugar, such as fresh fruit and complex carbohydrates. If you find cutting out sugar difficult or have cravings make sure you are eating enough protein – at every meal and snack is ideal. You can also supplement with fish oils, chromium and the herb gymnema as they assist insulin with the transportation of glucose, and mitigate the desire for sugar.

Caffeine. A little bit of caffeine is ok, but too much can increase the stress hormone cortisol. Studies also show that too much caffeine can trigger anxiety and lead to panic attacks.

Cutting back on caffeine is more likely to make you feel calmer, more relaxed and better overall mental health. PLUS it massively improves your sleep!

TAKE ACTION The best way is to remove caffeine slowly – not go cold turkey. You can start by swapping some of your caffeinated drinks for caffeine-free alternatives, like decaf, ginger tea, lemon tea or peppermint tea.

Alcohol. The link between alcohol and mental health is well documented. Alcohol is a depressant, which can disrupt the balance of neurotransmitters in your brain and affect your feelings, thoughts and behaviour – they key ones being serotonin and dopamine.

Cutting out alcohol can be hard, especially as it's often central in our social lives. But the benefits are game changing: increased energy, better mental clarity, better sleep, clearer skin, increased productivity and a stable mood.

TAKE ACTION My advice is to stick to low sugar drinks and make sure you drink a glass of water between each beverage.

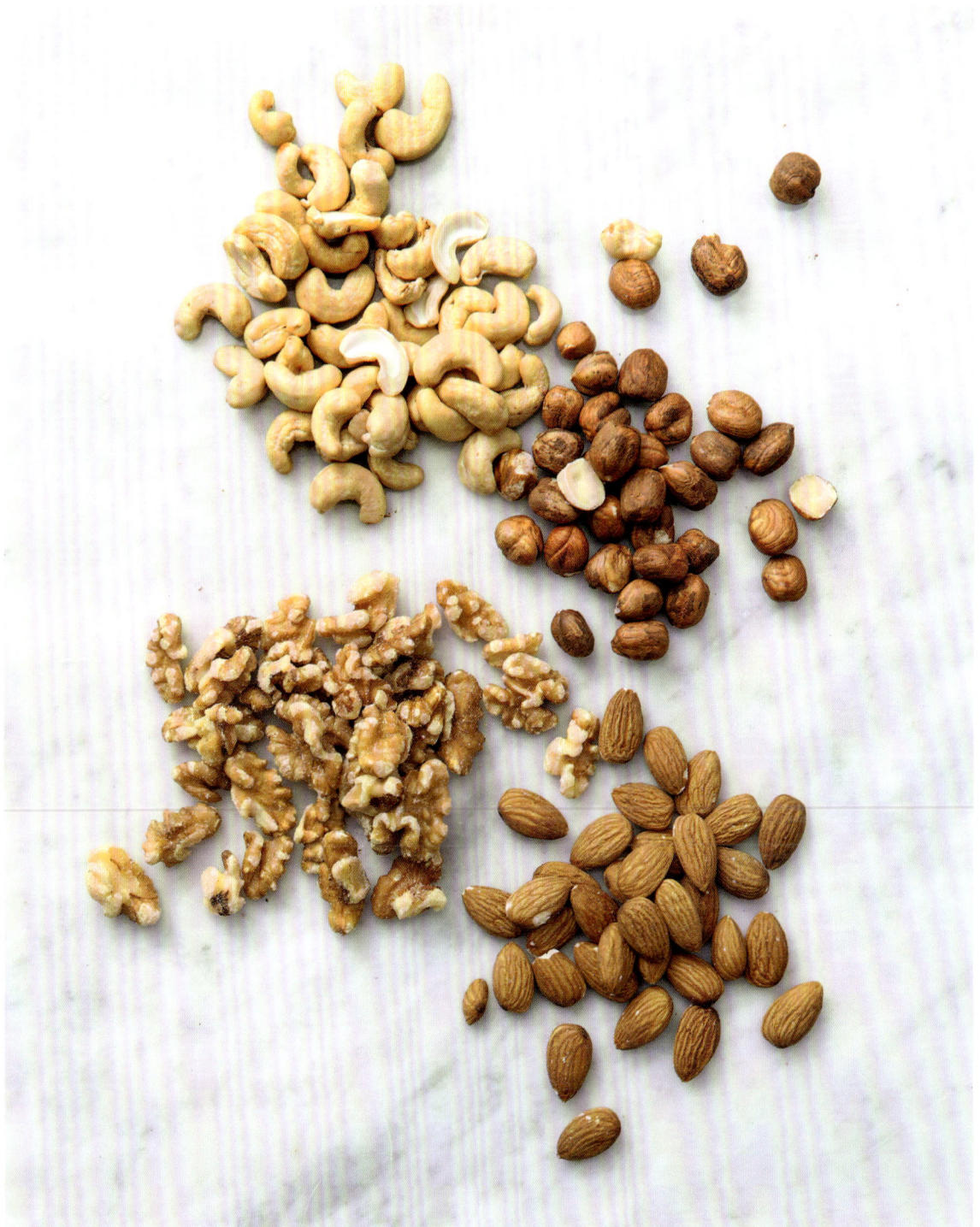

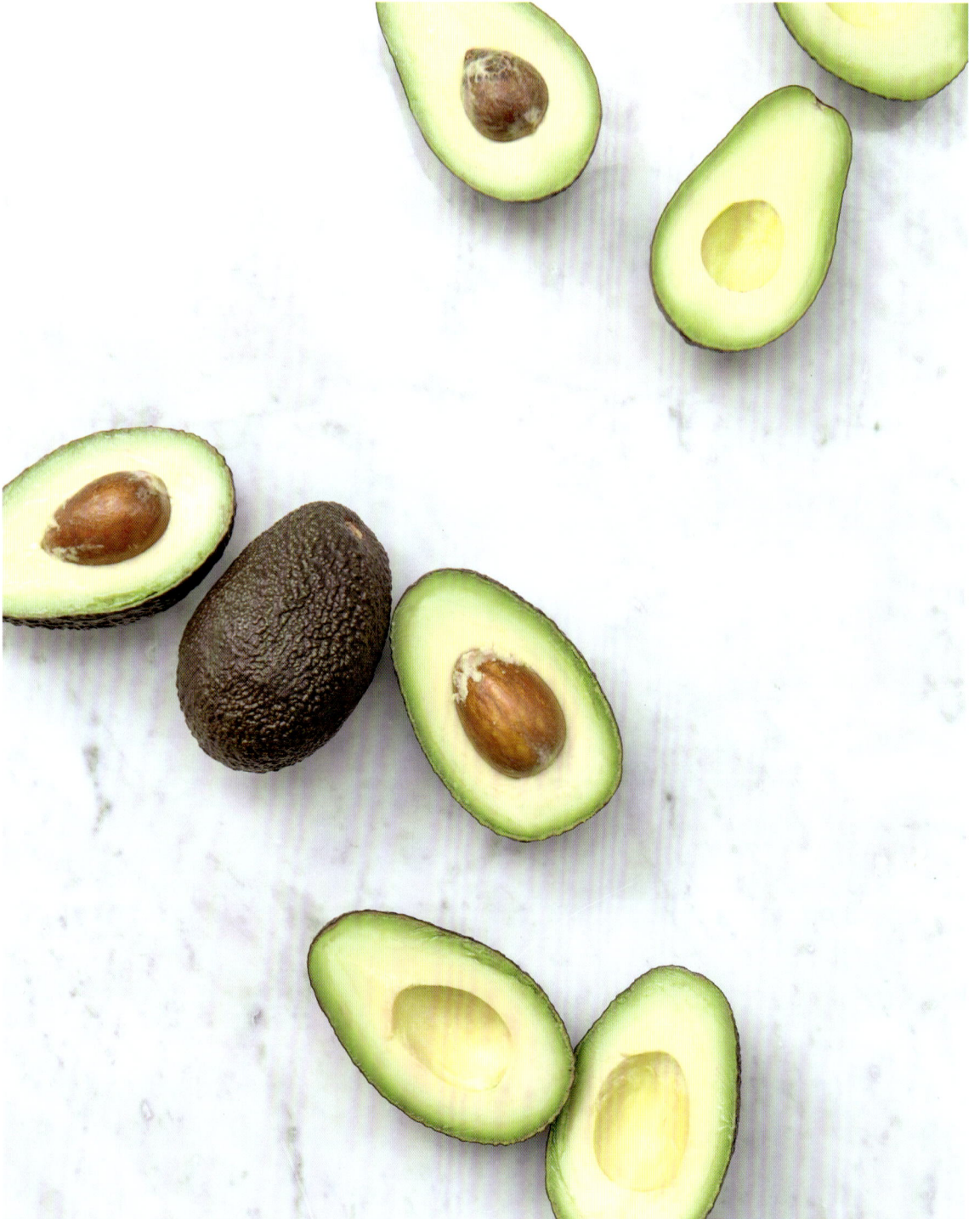

Foods to Increase to Feel Better

Protein. High protein foods such as chicken, fish, quinoa and lentils don't affect blood glucose (see page 42). They also contain an amino acid called tryptophan which gets converted into serotonin in the body – the happy hormone. Equally, the amino acid tyrosine helps the body produce dopamine. Tyrosine rich foods include chicken, turkey, fish, almonds, avocados, bananas, pumpkin seeds, and sesame seeds.

Fats. Your brain is 70% fat and the quality of fat you eat reflects the quality of fats in your brain. You brain needs fatty acids (such as omega-3 and -6) to keep it working well. Healthy fats are found in oily fish, poultry, nuts (especially walnuts and almonds), olive and sunflower oils, seeds (such as sunflower and pumpkin), avocados and eggs. Eat daily!

Depression and Inflammation

There is fascinating new evidence that now suggests that depression isn't solely down to low levels of serotonin. Several studies indicate that only 25 percent of depressed patients have low levels of the neurotransmitters serotonin and norepinephrine.

A large body of research now suggests that depression is associated with a low-grade, chronic inflammatory response, and is accompanied by increased oxidative stress. So, if you want to reduce depression and feel happy you have to reduce the inflammation in your brain and eat an anti-inflammatory diet.

Foods with anti-inflammatory properties include:

- Almonds
- Apples
- Avocados
- Berries
- Blueberries
- Brazil muts
- Broccoli
- Chamomile tea
- Chicken
- Dark chocolate
- Dark, leafy vegetables (spinach, cabbage)
- Eggs
- Kale
- Lentils
- Oily fish (salmon, trout, mackerel, herring, sardines)
- Rolled oats
- Sweet potatoes

How Does Caffeine Affect Energy?

Many of us rely on a cup of coffee or tea to wake us up, to keep us going through the morning and to provide a mid-afternoon boost. While this may appear a harmless habit, it is not the ideal solution to slumping energy levels and it can have a negative effect on our health.

Caffeine is a stimulant which can trigger the release of adrenaline and cortisol, providing the body with a quick burst of energy as it causes blood sugar levels to rise. This rise can also give the brain a boost and we may notice improvements in mood and alertness. However, this 'high' is soon followed by a slump, giving rise to dizziness, irritability, anxiety, sweating, palpitations, cravings (often for something sweet), poor concentration and the need for another pick-me-up. This rollercoaster leads to a reliance on greater amounts of caffeine and other stimulants.

The Health Implications of Caffeine

Caffeine is an 'anti-nutrient' which prevents the absorption of important vitamins and minerals and can also promote their excretion, including B vitamins, vitamin C, calcium, magnesium, zinc and iron – nutrients that are required for energy, immunity, stress management and cardiovascular and bone health.

Adrenaline and cortisol are stress hormones. In other words, when caffeine triggers their release, it is doing so by telling the adrenal glands to mount a stress response. A study published in 2005 found that drinking too much caffeine can contribute to sleep disorders and increase feelings of anxiety. Caffeine can also trigger the release of insulin if it is consumed continually, and high levels of insulin in the blood is how diabetes develops.

How Much is Too Much?

You can tell if you're drinking too much coffee because you will get the shakes. That jittery feeling means that your liver is not producing enough enzymes to break down the caffeine.

I'm usually happy for people to drink one cup of coffee per day but, while following my six-week programme, I want you to cut it out altogether so you can see how energized you become without this superficial energy supply. When I was recovering from burnout I cut out caffeine for a whole year and I can honestly say that my energy improved significantly.

The Gut-Brain Axis

The gut is the cornerstone to good health. When you have a healthy gut, you are most likely to feel well and happy. It's all down to the gut-brain 'axis', or the gut-brain connection. This is the biochemical signalling that takes place between the gastrointestinal tract and the central nervous system. The gut flora communicates with the brain via the vagus nerve which works in both directions – gut to brain, brain to gut.

The gut produces many of the neurotransmitters in our body, through the trillions of microbes living there. These are live bacteria that restore the gut and make you feel well. These powerful microorganisms generate 95% of the happy hormone serotonin and 50% of the pleasure hormone dopamine.

There is also a strong link between taking probiotics and improving your mood and mental wellbeing. A review of 15 human studies found supplementing with Bifidobacterium and Lactobacillus strains for 1–2 months can improve anxiety, depression, and memory, and help with autism and obsessive-compulsive disorder (OCD). Many studies also show a correlation between probiotics and lower levels of depression.

How to Improve Gut Health

- Increase your fibre with foods like legumes, beans, and fruit. Dietary fibre is fermented in the gut and produces short-chain fatty acids which strengthen the intestinal cells and help to reduce inflammation.

- Eat fermented foods such as yogurt, sauerkraut, miso and kombucha which all contain healthy bacteria and can reduce the number of disease-causing species in the gut.

- Eat prebiotic foods. Prebiotics are a type of fibre that stimulates the growth of healthy bacteria. They literally feed the friendly bacteria in the gut. Prebiotic rich foods include bananas, asparagus, oats and apples.

- Increase polyphenols, plant compounds that positively impact your gut because they are high in micronutrients. Try foods like green tea, ginger and mint.

- Avoid excessive amounts of highly-processed foods and added sugars. They can decrease the number of good bacteria and diversity in your gut.

- Take a probiotic daily, as they help your body to produce the happy hormones. But it's important to take a probiotic with multiple strains, so that it mimics the ecosystem in the gut.

What about Gluten?

Gluten is a protein found in certain grassy grains like wheat, barley and rye. It is the component that gives elasticity to dough, helping it rise and keep its shape, often giving the final product a chewy texture.

We all know that people with coeliac disease HAVE to remove gluten from their diets as it dramatically damages the gut lining. Now medical experts largely agree that there is a condition related to gluten sensitivity other than coeliac disease. Coeliac experts now use the term non-coeliac gluten sensitivity (NCGS) for those people who react to gluten without having coeliac disease. NCGS is when individuals experience symptoms similar to those of coeliac disease but do not have raised antibodies nor the damage to the intestines that coeliac patients have.

Should We All Avoid Gluten?

In the 10 years of my clinical practice I have witnessed that people not only seem to do better on a gluten-free diet – they thrive. I can honestly say that it almost always results in improved energy, weight loss, better digestion, clearer skin, less brain fog and better sleep. I'm not saying everyone should avoid gluten, but I have seen many people thrive when they remove it from their diet.

Are you Sensitive to Gluten?

Here are some signs to look out for:

> Weight loss or weight gain
> Nutritional deficiencies due to malabsorption, for example low iron levels
> Gastrointestinal problems (bloating, pain, gas, constipation, diarrhoea)
> Fatigue after eating
> Aching joints
> Depression
> Eczema
> Headaches
> Exhaustion

Foods that Contain Gluten

> Bread
> Pasta
> Biscuits
> Cakes
> Bulgur wheat
> Couscous
> Egg noodles
> Rye
> Spelt
> Durum flour
> Kamut
> Semolina

How to Follow a Gluten-free Diet

Bread and pasta are the most common wheat and gluten products, but when following a gluten-free diet it is important to remember that gluten is also found in most biscuits, cakes, cereals, sausages, pies and a surprising number of sauces.

Fortunately, all food products have to disclose the exact content of their ingredients, no matter how small the amount. Therefore, by checking the label, you can assure yourself you are avoiding even the tiniest amount of gluten.

Embarking on a gluten-free diet may seem daunting but with a little preparation, and the abundance of gluten-free products available on the market, the change can be achievable and hopefully beneficial.

There are many naturally gluten-free foods that you can choose from, such as lentils, chickpeas, rice, quinoa, beans and corn. You can also look for alternatives such as rice pasta, quinoa bread, rice cakes and noodles etc. Most supermarkets have a section of gluten-free products including breads, biscuits, pastas and pizza bases. But please check the ingredients. As a rule of thumb, if you can't pronounce it, don't eat it!

My six-week meal plan is completely gluten free so you can follow the plan and hopefully notice changes in your energy levels.

How Many Calories Should I be Eating?

Too often I see men and women in my clinic not eating enough and overexercising. Cringe! I get so nervous when I see it as this alone is a recipe for burnout.

Ladies, you need to consume 2,000 calories per day. Guys, you need to consume around 2,500 calories per day. And if you are active, add another 500–1,000 calories.

If we reduce our calorie intake it really affects our energy so, for now, while you are recovering, I want you to focus on more food going in. If you are eating the right foods and not overeating then you will not put on weight. If you want to monitor your calorie intake, I recommend using an app such as MyFitnessPal which shows your daily intake as well as the macronutrient ratios.

What about Dairy?

Milk and dairy products are usually cited as an essential part of the human diet due to their high levels of calcium. It is undoubtedly true that dairy products are packed with nutrients, but this does not mean that the combination of nutrients in dairy products is suited to human nutrition. The best diet for any species must be the one to which it is genetically adapted. Archaeological studies show that humans started to selectively breed animals for their milk around 2,000 years ago. This is too short a time for our digestive systems to have adapted.

Approximately 65 per cent of the world's population has some difficulty digesting lactose after infancy. This is why many cultures around the world do not eat dairy. After infancy, most humans do not naturally produce enough lactase, the enzyme required to metabolize the milk sugar lactose. And without lactase, the lactose ferments in the intestines, causing abdominal discomfort, excessive gas, bloating, cramping, diarrhoea and irritable bowel syndrome. Not nice.

Having said that, I'm okay with some dairy in the diet because it is a good source of protein and it's packed with other nutrients such as vitamin D, A, B12 and folate.

And so I would say: if you do suffer from any of the symptoms listed above, try cutting out dairy for two weeks. You can then reintroduce it and notice whether your symptoms come back. You might find that you are much happier eating less or no dairy.

It's important to remember that when you take something out of your diet it's a good idea to replace it with something else. In this case try swapping cows' yogurt for soya yogurt, for example.

Dairy Allergy or Intolerance?

An allergy occurs when the immune system reacts to the proteins found in milk. The body reacts to the proteins as if they are a harmful substance. Children are most prone to dairy allergy but anyone can be affected at any time in their life. Symptoms of a dairy allergy can occur very quickly and include skin rash, digestive upsets, vomiting, bloating and stomach cramps.

The most common reason for needing to avoid dairy products is an intolerance to lactose, the natural sugar in milk. It usually happens because the body can't produce enough of the enzyme lactase to aid proper digestion. Lactose intolerance produces symptoms similar to a mild allergy. It can be quite difficult to diagnose, as symptoms often occur some hours after consuming dairy.

What about Calcium?

We do need calcium for healthy bones but not necessarily from dairy sources. The good news is it's really easy to go dairy free now. There are plenty of products out there that cater for a dairy-free diet, including many plant-based milks.

We can also obtain calcium from other wholefood sources, like dark green leafy vegetables, sesame tahini, almonds, soybean products, dried fruits (especially figs), sea vegetables and tinned salmon or sardines with the bones left in. And so if you are cutting dairy out of your diet, make sure you are getting calcium from other foods.

The Importance of Protein

I'm ALWAYS harping on about protein because it is really important for energy management, the production of many hormones, including cortisol (remember, cortisol is essential to the proper functioning of the body, we just don't want to constantly trigger its release unnecessarily), supporting recovery and much more. Protein foods are also made up of essential amino acids (see opposite), which are vital for our bodies to function.

You need a gram of protein each day per kilogram of body weight. So, if you weigh 60kg (132lb) you need to eat 60g (2oz) of protein each day. If you weigh 80kg (176lb) you need to eat 80g (nearly 3oz) of protein. One egg only gives you 7g (¼oz) of protein, a 100g (3½oz) chicken breast gives you 30g (1oz) of protein, and a 100g (3½oz) fish fillet gives you 25g (¾oz) of protein.

My advice is to eat protein at every meal and snack.

Can You Have Too Much?

Most research indicates that eating more than 2g of protein per kilogram (about 2¼ lb) of body weight – that's double the recommended amount – over a long period of time can cause health problems, mostly to the kidneys.

Which Foods Contain Protein?

The following are good-quality protein sources that I want you to focus on.

> Chicken
> Fish
> Lean meat
> Eggs
> Quinoa
> Chickpeas
> Lentils
> Tofu
> Protein powders

What are Amino Acids?

Amino acids are the building blocks the body relies on to function. They are required for manufacturing hormones, building muscle and regulating our immune system. They are also important for improving our mood and sleep.

There are nine amino acids that we call 'essential' because our bodies do not make them. This means we need to ingest them. When we eat protein foods, they get broken down by enzymes in the body into amino acids. That is why it is so important to eat protein foods.

Five Signs you are Lacking Protein

1. **You have low energy and suffer from fatigue.** You need to be eating protein at every meal and snack to keep your blood sugar levels on a nice even keel to provide you with sustainable energy every day.

2. **You have food cravings.** Protein takes four hours to break down in the gut and keeps us feeling full. If you are not eating protein regularly, it can lead to cravings. Protein can prevent blood sugar spikes and dips.

3. **Your muscles feel weak and you have poor workout recovery.** Everyone knows that protein is needed to build new muscle mass. A low-protein diet can result in muscle wasting.

4. **You have thin hair and weak nails.** If you want super strong and healthy hair and nails, it's all about the protein. It's literally food for hair and nails.

5. **You feel anxious and moody.** Amino acids are the building blocks of neurotransmitters and hormones that control your mood, including dopamine and serotonin which help bring on positive feelings such as calm, excitement and positivity.

What about Protein Powders?

Protein powders provide a quick and efficient way of getting much-needed protein into the body, and I often use them in breakfast smoothies to kick-start my day.

There are lots of different types of protein powders. The most common are whey protein, rice, pea, hemp and soya.

You want to make sure you have a protein powder which provides at least 20g (¾ oz) of protein per serving. You can purchase protein powders with additional vitamins and minerals but look out for added ingredients that are not beneficial to the body. Some protein powders include many other ingredients such as sweeteners, artificial flavours and thickeners, so make sure you read the label before you buy. Again, as a rule of thumb, if you can't pronounce it, don't eat it!

You can buy good brands from reputable health stores. If buying online, stick to more boutique brands, as the ingredients and quality tends to be much better. If possible, I would advise changing up your protein powders to make sure you are getting a variety of proteins in your diet. But if you are suffering with digestive complaints then choose a dairy-free version and go for a rice protein, as they are the easiest to digest.

Chapter Four

Choosing Supplements

Everything is important until you're sick, then you realise there was only one thing that was important. Your health.

Nutrients play a key role in keeping us healthy. Of course, it's preferable to get our vitamins and minerals from our food but in my work I see a lot of nutrient deficiencies. In fact, an estimated 2 billion people have at least one nutrient deficiency globally, and the most common are iron, vitamin D, B12 and magnesium. A massive 50% of the population of the US is deficient in magnesium alone!

This is where supplementation can be used as part of your energy toolkit.

As the name suggests, they are supplements to your diet, meaning you should be able to get most of the vitamins and minerals you need from your diet alone. However, since modern living can take its toll on the levels of some nutrients in your tissues, then supplementation – when used correctly – can be effective.

As a nutritionist, part of my job is identifying which nutrients clients may or may not be deficient in. I've been recommending supplements to clients for ten years now and here's my lowdown on them.

I never take a blanket approach to supplements with my clients. I always run tests before I make any recommendations.

TAKE ACTION
Blood tests are a good place to start, so book an appointment with your doctor.

'The supplement industry is a minefield. I can help you to navigate the supplement aisle'

Blood Tests for Deficiencies

The first thing I always look at is the blood. If you are lacking in energy, I recommend you get an appointment with your doctor right away to test your levels of iron, vitamin B12, vitamin D and thyroid hormones.

Iron

Iron is a mineral which carries out many functions in the body. Iron is part of haemoglobin, the protein that carries oxygen in the bloodstream to all of the organs in the body. If you are lacking in iron, you are likely to feel fatigued, dizzy, weak, have headaches, have cold hands and feet, suffer shortness of breath (even after walking up some stairs), difficulty concentrating, hair loss, brittle nails and pale skin.

Before you start to supplement iron, however, please get your levels tested as too much iron in the body can lead to haemochromatosis, which can kill you. So get it tested.

If your iron levels are found to be low, you can eat more iron-rich foods such as red meat, fish, beans, tofu, eggs and green leafy vegetables including kale, broccoli and spinach. You can also take iron supplements but be careful which type of iron you take. For example, you want to make sure that the iron is chelated. Chelated iron has been chemically altered to allow it to pass through the digestive tract. Choose the supplements which have

iron bisglycinate or iron chelate because they are better absorbed and less toxic in the body. Non-chelated iron can cause constipation.

Another thing to remember: vitamin C massively helps the absorption of iron. So eat foods rich in vitamin C when taking iron supplements or eating iron-rich foods. Good choices are strawberries, oranges, blueberries, red peppers, tomatoes and butternut squash.

Vitamin B12

Vitamin B12 is one of the most important vitamins for promoting energy. This is because it's involved in the production of ATP (Adenosine triphosphate), which is vital for energy transfer within cells. If there's not enough B12 present at a cellular level, ATP will not be produced. If you are lacking in B12 you may feel tired, weak, light headed, have a shortness of breath and pale skin.

Your body cannot produce B12, which is why you have to ingest it. It is found predominantly in animal produce such as beef, chicken, trout, salmon, tuna and eggs, as well as fortified cereals.

You can also get injections of B12 if your levels are low or you can take supplements, but have a blood test first to check whether you are deficient. The NHS recommends a daily intake of 1.5 micrograms (mcg) for adults aged 19 to 64.

Vitamin D

Vitamin D actually acts more like a hormone and every single cell in your body has a receptor for it. It's required for so many things, such as regulating calcium, building healthy bones, strengthening the immune system and reducing inflammation.

How do you tell if you're lacking vitamin D? Here are my top four most common signs and symptoms.

1. **Fatigue and tiredness.** Very low levels of vitamin D can actually cause extreme fatigue so it's definitely worth getting a blood test.

2. **Getting sick often.** Vitamin D helps to regulate the immune system so if you don't have enough then you could be getting every cold going.

3. **Weak bones.** Vitamin D is needed for building osteoblasts (cells that secrete the substance of bone) so you may feel that your bones are weak or that they are not as strong as they used to be.

4. **Depression.** This is a big one. Research shows there is a link between vitamin D deficiency and depression.

Getting vitamin D from your food is quite hard as few foods contain significant amounts, so injections and supplements are more effective. If supplementing, choose vitamin D3 which is the active form. Some supplements on the market only provide vitamin D2 which is the inactive form. A daily vitamin D intake of 1,000–4,000 international units (iu) or 25–100mcg should be enough to ensure optimal blood levels for most people. Again, get your levels tested by a doctor before you look to supplements.

But the easiest way to get more vitamin D is to sit in the sun. Sitting in the sun for 20 minutes provides you with 20,000iu of vitamin D. It's actually synthesized in the skin. Please note that wearing sunscreen negates this, but you should always wear sunscreen if you are being exposed to the sun in the middle of the day.

'Make sure you get your vitamin levels tested by a doctor before you look to supplements'

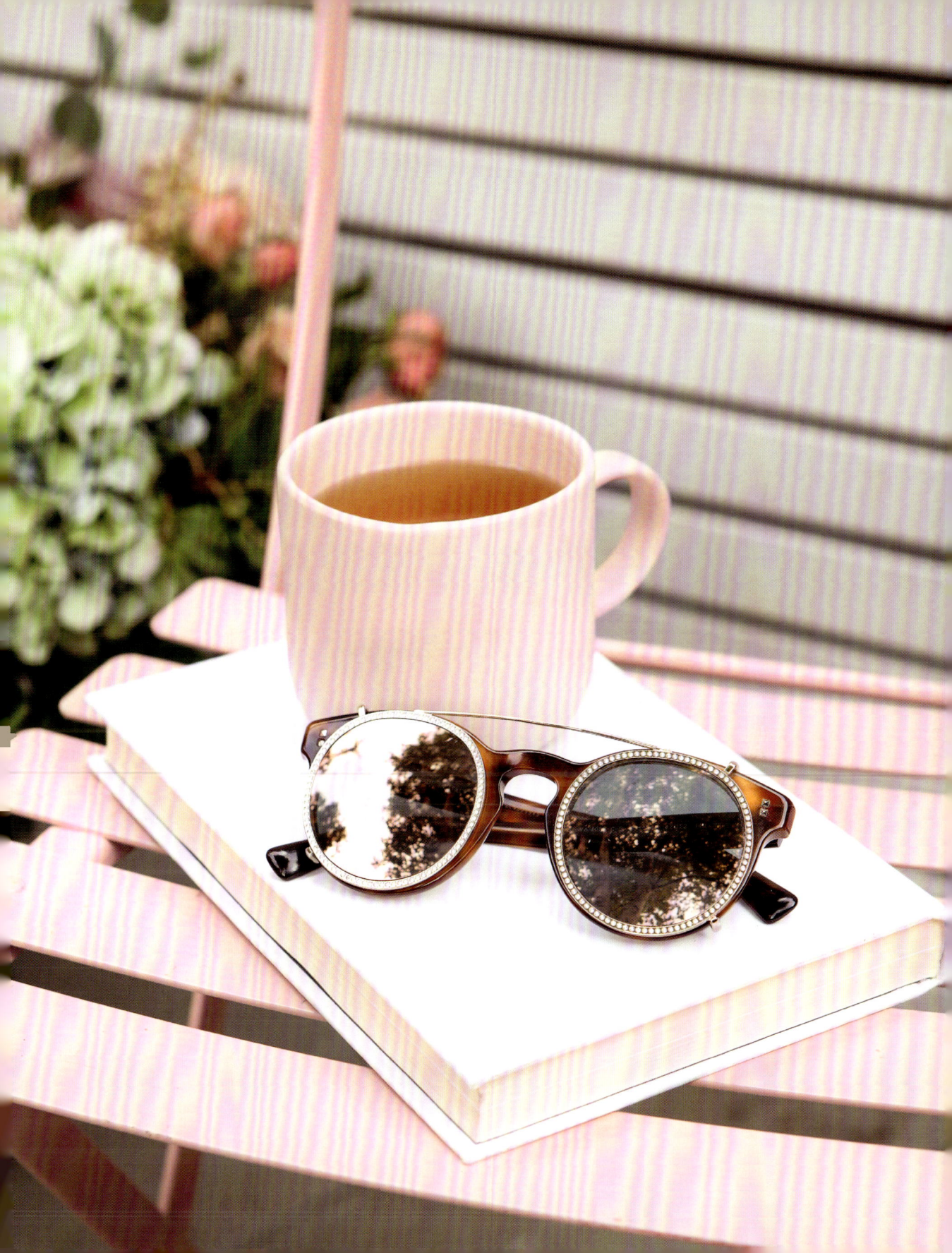

Thyroid Testing

The thyroid gland is situated just below the Adam's apple in the neck. It is fairly small, normally weighing around 25g (1oz), but is solely responsible for running your body's metabolism. If your thyroid gland is not working efficiently then you are likely to experience the following symptoms:

– Fatigue

– Energy drops in the afternoon

– Feeling better when exposed to sunshine

– Feeling cold easily

– Tiredness and sleeping a lot

– Dry and/or pale skin

– Coarse, thinning hair and brittle nails

– Sore muscles, slow movements and weakness

– A hoarse or croaky voice

– Depression

– Problems with memory and concentration

– Weight gain

– Digestive issues

TAKE ACTION
If you feel like you resonate with these signs and symptoms, here are some other questions to ask yourself:

– Are your energy levels lower than they were five years ago?

– Is your concentration worse than it was five years ago?

– Is your short-term memory declining?

– Do you experience aches and pains or stiffness in your muscles and joints?

– Do you feel at your worst mid-afternoon?

– Are you someone who is always cold?

– Do you suffer any digestive problems or constipation?

– Do you have high cholesterol?

– Has your sex drive plummeted?

– Are you a stressful person?

If you answered yes to any of these questions then it's definitely time to get your thyroid tested with a blood test.

TAKE ACTION

If you do have an underactive thyroid then the doctor is likely to recommend thyroxine medication but you can consider easing your symptoms by trying the following:

1. Limit your consumption of goitrogenic foods such as broccoli, Brussels sprouts, cabbage, cauliflower, kale, turnips, peaches, peanuts, radishes, soybeans, spinach and strawberries. Goitrogens are compounds found in these foods which can interfere with thyroid function. Cooking does appear to help inactivate the goitrogenic compounds, so if you are going to eat these foods it would be wise to eat them cooked rather than raw.

2. Drink filtered water as the chlorine and fluoride in tap water can compete with iodine which is an extremely important mineral for thyroid hormone production.

3. Increase your intake of foods rich in iodine such as kelp, fish and dulse seaweed. Iodine is a mineral that is needed to manufacture the thyroid hormones thyroxine (T4) and triiodothyronine (T3).

4. Selenium is also essential for a healthy thyroid. The enzyme that converts thyroid hormone T4 into the more physiologically active hormone T3 contains selenium. Without it, this conversion cannot take place, resulting in an underactive thyroid gland. Good sources of selenium include Brazil nuts, eggs, tuna and chicken.

Hair Mineral Testing

I really like using hair mineral analysis tests. I use them on my clients because they measure mineral deficiencies in the body's tissues, as well as heavy metal toxicity. Just by sending a small sample of your hair to a lab they can identify mineral deficiencies and find the most likely causes. Good companies usually provide you with a detailed and comprehensive report which explains which foods you need to eat and avoid, as well as which supplements you need to take to get your levels back up again.

TAKE ACTION
If you're interested in understanding more about your deficiencies, go to a website such as www.mineralcheck.com and check the tests that they offer. They will send you a kit and you send it back to the lab for testing. If you're after a specific and tailored nutrition and supplement plan, then this is for you.

Cortisol Testing

You can measure your 'live' cortisol levels with a saliva test. I have used this test hundreds of times in my clinic to give an insight into what is going on physiologically. This test is not diagnostic but does give a snapshot into what your adrenal glands are doing on that day and to see how much stress is affecting you.

Typically your cortisol levels should be high in the morning, decline throughout the day and be the lowest at night. High levels of cortisol in the morning motivate you to get out of bed. As it gets darker, the pineal gland in the back of the brain releases melatonin, the hormone that gets you ready for bed. With a cortisol test you have to take four saliva samples throughout the day – one in the morning, one midday, one mid-afternoon and one just before you sleep – and send them off to a lab for testing. They will send you a copy of your results with a breakdown of the readings.

TAKE ACTION
This test is not diagnostic but provides a window of identification. It is very simple to do in the comfort of your own home and relatively inexpensive. However, you do need a healthcare practitioner such as a nutritionist or chiropractor to request the test for you.

Ragland's Blood Pressure Test

This is a simple test to measure your blood pressure and determine the level of adrenal health and function. You will need a blood pressure machine for this test, which can be done in the comfort of your own home.

TAKE ACTION

1. Lie down with a blood pressure monitor on your arm. Rest for 5 minutes then take a blood pressure reading.

2. Stand up and take your blood pressure again.

Normal blood pressure is around 120 over 80. The systolic blood pressure (the number on the top) should rise by 8–10mm after standing up. If your number doesn't rise, or if it drops by 8–10mm or more, this could indicate that your adrenal glands are struggling.

Salts, Blood Pressure and Dizziness

One thing I really want to highlight to you is that in my experience people who are suffering from burnout typically have low blood pressure. If you test your blood pressure and your readings come up on the low side, you may benefit from more salt in your diet.

You can start by adding a little more salt to your food, or drink half a teaspoon of rock salt in a glass of water first thing each morning. It helps to lift you, raise blood pressure and can stop feelings of dizziness. I like using pink Himalayan salt.

Which Nutrients Give You Energy?

Many nutrients are required to maintain cellular energy, but three stand out from the crowd because they are absolutely crucial, especially if you have burnout. They are:

Siberian Ginseng

This is an adaptogenic herb, so whatever your cortisol levels are doing, this supplement can help to bring them back into balance. Research published in the *Journal of Ginseng Research* in 2017 suggests that Siberian ginseng aids may help to reduce some of the negative effects of stress. This herb is also believed by many to support the adrenal glands, increase energy and enhance mental clarity. If you do take this supplement, take one at breakfast and one at lunchtime and try to avoid it in the afternoon because it can be quite stimulating.

B Vitamins

B Vitamins, particularly B1, B3, B5 and B12 (see page 61), help convert food into energy. They are essential in the production of ATP (Adenosine triphosphate), your body's energy molecule. If they are not present in the cells where ATP is made, you will not manufacture it, leaving you feeling tired. B vitamins work better in synergy so it's best to take a B vitamin complex rather than taking a single B vitamin on its own.

Magnesium

Magnesium is a major muscle relaxant because it makes the blood vessels dilate, improving blood flow and allowing nutrients to travel in the blood more freely to where they are needed in the body. I recommend this nutrient if you're feeling tired but wired, particularly at night when you can't sleep. Adults can take supplements of up to 400mg of magnesium per day, or you can put it in your bath in the form of Epsom bath salts. You can order these in bulk really cheaply online. Simply sprinkle into a warm bath and soak for 20 minutes.

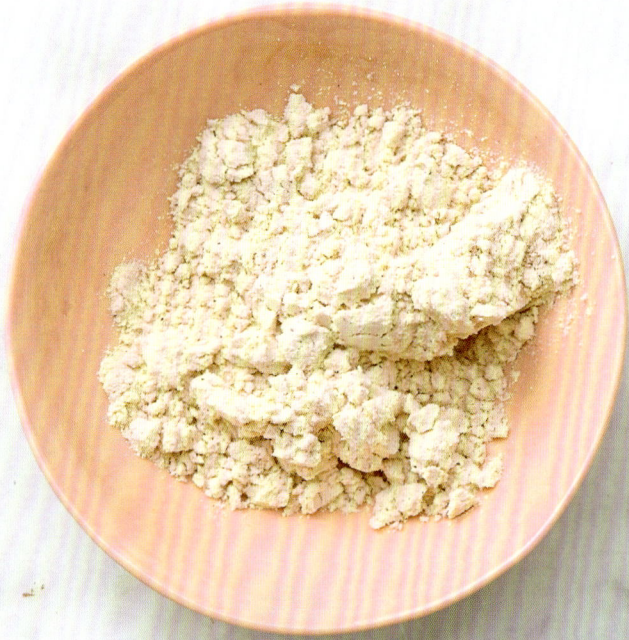

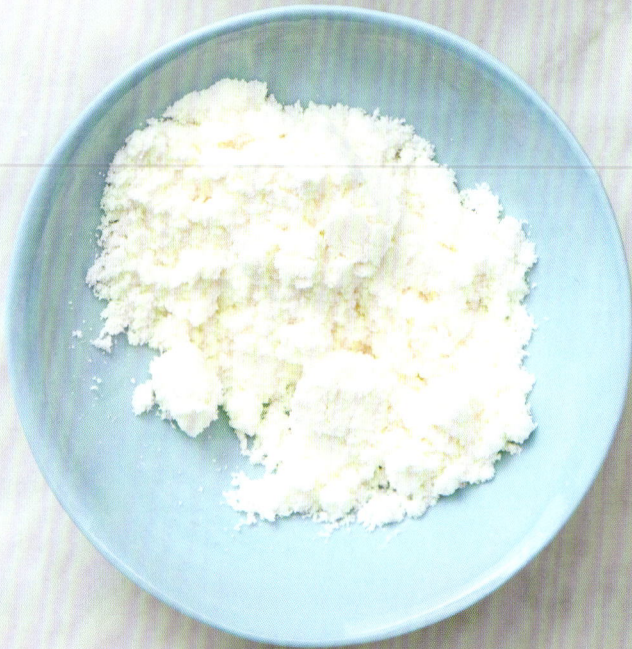

How To Choose a Good Probiotic

Probiotics are live bacteria and yeasts, and are great for gut health (see page 51). I recommend taking a daily probiotic if you're struggling with your gut and mental health. Here are some tips on what to look out for when choosing yours:

1. Choose the right strains for you. Different strains do different things. Once you know the name of the strain, you can see what it's been researched for and use those cultures according to your needs. For example, Bifidobacterium helps to reduce depression whilst Lactobacillus rhamnosus is good for helping with anxiety.

2. Go for a product with multiple strains, as this is more likely to mimic the microbes in your gut.

3. Make sure the supplement you choose has an effective dose. It's important to look for probiotics that contain at least 10^6 (i.e. 1 million) CFUs (Colony Forming Units) per gram, as research suggests that this is the minimum amount needed to exert positive effects in the body.

4. Choose a trusted brand. There are SO many products on the market. Make sure you go for a specialist brand with products that have been backed by sound science.

Where to Get Supplements

You do get what you pay for when it comes to supplements so make sure you get yours from reputable companies. They are likely to care about your health and the products they stock are of better quality.

Be careful of the supplements available in pharmacy chain stores because the bioavailability (absorption rate) can be poor, the dosages tend to be a lot lower and they are often packed with fillers and preservatives such as caking agents. Here are my top tips for choosing supplements:

1. Avoid minerals in the form of oxides, sulphates and carbonates, which are difficult for your body to absorb. Choose those in the form of citrates instead.

2. Choose a natural form of vitamin E (d-alpha-tocopherol) rather than the synthetic version (dl-alpha-tocopherol), which is not so easily absorbed.

3. Choose vitamin B6 as pyridoxal-5-phosphate, not the cheaper pyridoxine, as it is easier for your body to use.

4. Buy vitamin D as D3 cholecalciferol, not D2 ergocalciferol, as D3 is the active form and is more effective at raising and maintaining levels.

5. Take vitamin C as an ascorbate rather than ascorbic acid.

6. When buying fish oils, make sure the ratios of EPA and DHA are at the optimal level of

2:1. Avoid cod liver oils which are extracted from the liver of the fish rather than the body of the fish, as the liver may contain toxins and heavy metals such as mercury.

7. If taking iron supplements, be aware that some can be constipating. The best form of iron that does not cause constipation is iron bisglycinate.

8. When choosing probiotics, avoid those in yogurt-based products as these are usually loaded with sugar. It's best to get either powdered or capsule versions. Choose a product with both bioacidophillus and bifodobacterium as these are the strains which have the most human studies supporting their benefits. You want to purchase a probiotic which has at least 22 billion microorganisms in total. Watch out for products containing maltodextrin as this is a sugar which can lead to blood sugar fluctuations. Instead go for probiotics with FOS (fructooligosaccharides). These are prebiotics and help to feed the existing friendly bacteria in your gut.

9. Silicon dioxide can be found in many supplements and is used as an anti-caking agent to prevent foods from absorbing moisture and clumping together. No scientific research has suggested it is a necessary nutrient for our bodies, nor has research found any sign that it causes harm. It's up to you whether you choose a product with or without it.

To Do

1. First things first, get a blood test done. Whether that means booking an appointment with your doctor or using a private service, I don't mind – just get your nutrient levels measured, particularly for iron, vitamin D, vitamin B12 and your thyroid.

2. Take a look at your existing supplement programme and decide which ones you can continue taking and which ones can be paused for now.

3. Take the hair mineral analysis test and identify which nutrients your tissues are actually deficient in. If you're really serious about doing whatever it takes to get your energy back, this step is key for you.

Chapter Five

Lifestyle Changes

'You're not burned out because you're doing too much, you're burned out because you're doing too little of what makes you feel alive. '

If you really want to get to the bottom of your fatigue, this chapter may blow your mind. I explain all of the unexpected reasons you could be tired all the time, giving you the insight to make some significant changes and move forward. Most of these reasons are things that you may have overlooked, so I think you're going be really surprised.

Wanna know the number one reason you're tired all the time...?

You're Doing Too Much!

Fatigue often hits when your plate is already full but you keep adding to it. It's true, right? We've all been there – we say yes to everything and knowingly take on too much. And after the workload, we still have to fit in errands, find time to exercise, go out and be social, spend time with loved ones, maintain the kids' agendas...the list goes on.

Most of us take on more than we can manage and gradually our workload and to-do lists keep growing, never getting smaller. Well let me tell you something – this is the fastest way to feel overwhelmed. But often we feel overwhelmed due to a lack of prioritizing. Feeling frazzled usually comes down to poor organization and time management. PLUS we are so distracted these days. Sit down for five minutes and your phone will show at least five notifications. The average person taps and swipes on their phone thousands of times a day.

TAKE ACTION

But where do we draw the line? How do we reduce the feelings of being overwhelmed?

Here are my top tips for you:

1. **Prioritize.** Look at your list of things to do and identify the three things that are urgent or most important. Focus only on those until they are done. Ask yourself what things you need to do in order to move the needle on them. And then, when they are complete, write down the next three tasks.

2. **Cut back.** You don't have to take on the world. I bet you could look at your to-do list and cut back on at least half. How many items are important but not really urgent? How many are not urgent and not important? Try writing a 'STOP DOING' list. Once you do you will feel a rush of relief and suddenly have a lot of time back.

3. **Delegate.** I love this one. And it's so overlooked. Just a gentle reminder that you don't have to do everything yourself. Don't be afraid to ask for help. Hand over tasks. Get your partner to do the cooking. What one thing can you offload and give to someone else? This is a great way to free up a bit more time. It's not your job to be everything to everyone. There are people who would LOVE to do your cleaning and ironing.

4. **Learn to say no without explaining yourself.** This is a big one and difficult to do but majorly powerful. As a rule of thumb, if it ain't a 'hell yeah!' it's a 'no'. So with that in mind, stop doing all the things you hate. Say no to them and don't feel bad about it. As long as you say no in a polite way then people will understand. PLUS the world will still go round.

   Here's how you can gently turn something down: 'Hi xxxx, Thank you so much for your request. I'd love to support you but at this moment in time I have a lot on my plate, most of which has been in the pipeline for over a year, and I wouldn't want to take something on without giving it my full attention. Would it be okay to get back in touch in six months?' See how easy that is?

5. **Slow down.** Slooooowwwww doooown. Think about how often you are rushing in your life. The commute, running errands, rushing to meetings, heading home after work, when you're driving. NO! Take your time. I urge you to identify the things you are always rushing and make the following changes:

   1. Give yourself five minutes more to do everything.

   2. Identify one thing that you do in a rushed state and slow down with it.

   For me it was when I walked anywhere. I literally had a Monday morning pace even on a Sunday. Now I make sure I leave a little extra time so I can walk a little slower, not climb up and down the escalators at the train station, and remind myself to breathe and be calm. What is yours going to be?

6. **Take a break at work.** Please, please, please take a break at work, and for goodness' sake, take your full hour for lunch. You are entitled to do so. At the very least, step outside of the office for half an hour. Eating your lunch at your desk will not boost your spirits or your energy levels.

7. **Interrupt the stress response.** Next time you feel you can't cope, step away from the situation. Like...literally. I want you to go outside for five minutes, breathe slowly and deeply, put everything into perspective, reset your intention and go back in. If you can't go outside, then look out the window as far as your eyes can see. Take in the view. It will change your perspective instantly.

Not Enough Sleep?

This is such a massive subject and it's so critical for energy. If you are not sleeping, you will not recover. End of. So why is sleep so important?

When we are sleeping, our bodies are hard at work repairing damage caused by stress. Our cells produce more protein while we are sleeping, and these protein molecules form the building blocks for our cells (see page 56). What's more, a study published in 2001 found a correlation between people with insomnia or interrupted sleep and elevated cortisol in the blood. That's right. The stress hormone.

One thing to point out is that the hours of sleep you get between 10pm and midnight are the most boosting. The theory is because when the sun goes down and it becomes dark, the pineal gland at the back of your brain releases a surge of melatonin. This is the natural hormone that makes you feel tired and helps you to fall asleep. During these hours it's considered to be the deepest and most regenerative sleep.

Adults between the age of 26 and 64 need 7–9 hours of sleep per night. Skimping on sleep and surviving on less than this is not a badge of honour. It will catch up with you sooner or later.

I can't emphasize the importance of sleep for recovery enough. To recover your energy you seriously need it. Please make this your upmost priority during the six-week plan.

TAKE ACTION
I understand that there are many insomniacs out there, so here are my top tips for getting a good night's sleep:

Routine. It's really important to stick to a routine when it comes to sleep. If you go to bed at the same time every night and wake up at the same time every morning, you are much more likely to have a healthy sleep/wake cycle. When we abuse our sleep routine, our energy levels start to suffer. Start setting up a good routine by going to bed earlier – even by just 30 minutes at a time – so that your body slowly gets used to it, and then build from there.

Light and darkness. When the sun goes down and it becomes dark, our pineal gland at the back of our head releases melatonin. If we are exposed to light in the evenings when we are meant to be winding down, this can really interfere with the natural release of melatonin. Be extra careful about the blue light from your phone, as research shows that too much blue light prevents the release of melatonin and reduces the feeling of alertness in the morning. So make sure you are sleeping in a dark room without access to blue light.

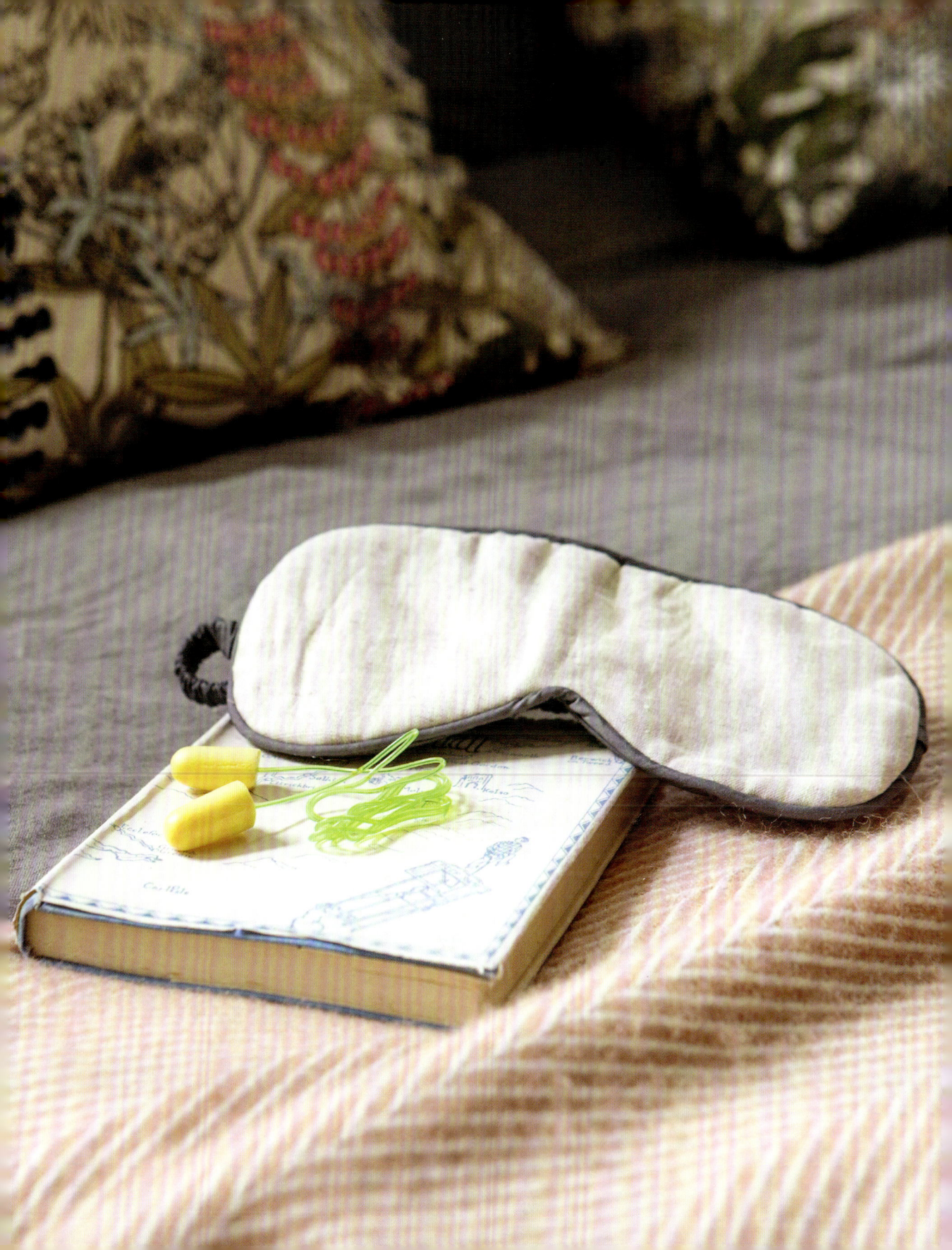

Temperature. Our body's temperature at night plays an important role when we are falling asleep. A review published in the *Journal of Physiological Anthropology* found that too much heat at night increases wakefulness and decreases our chances of REM (rapid eye movement) sleep – in other words, deep and restful sleep. So make sure you are in a cool room and not covered in too many clothes and covers!

Flight mode. This is an absolute game changer. Putting your phone on flight mode from 10pm until 6am will stop most of the distractions. You won't be on your phone scrolling through Instagram and you are less likely to pick up your phone again, knowing that you've deliberately put it on flight mode. If this isn't enough, put your phone out of reach under the bed, in a drawer or in another room so you are not tempted to grab it. One in three people check their phone in the middle of the night. Don't be one of the statistics.

Dim down. It's really important to 'dim down' an hour before you go to bed. This means putting your phone away and starting the routine of getting ready for bed. That might mean having a cup of chamomile tea, having a bath, doing some yoga – anything to tell the body you are getting ready for sleep.

Avoid alcohol. It massively disrupts sleep and is likely to wake you up in the middle of the night, multiple times, and affect your chances of deep REM sleep.

No caffeine! It's a stimulant and keeps you awake. It also affects the amount of deep REM sleep you get. No caffeine after 2pm please. You can do this.

CBD hemp oil. A growing body of scientific research suggests that CBD (cannabidiol) oil appears to ease anxiety, making it easier to fall asleep. It helps to lessen the mind chatter so that you can fall asleep faster. You can buy it in capsules or as an oil.

Ear plugs. Another game changer in the sleep arena. Ear plugs are excellent for blocking out noise that might be keeping you awake. The best ones are the silicone ones. If you have a partner who snores, these are definitely going to change your life. I can't sleep without them.

Make sure you're comfortable. Being comfortable in bed can make all the difference when it comes to getting a good night's sleep. Is it time to change your pillows? Do you know how old your mattress is? It might also be worth investing in a more luxurious duvet, duvet cover or other bedcover. One of my secrets to good sleep is a mattress topper, as they add an extra layer of comfort. They are extremely soft and are an excellent addition if you have a hard mattress that you are not yet ready to replace.

Reading. Reading before bed can help lower levels of stress. This is because, when reading a good book, your mind is distracted from the daily stresses and worries that cause tension. Is it time to find a good book? What was the last thing you read that you really enjoyed? What other titles are there that are similar that you might enjoy?

Meditation. There have been so many clinical trials documenting the positive effects of meditation on the body. It helps to calm down the body and take you away from 'fight or flight' mode. I really like apps such as Headspace, Calm and Buddhify – they help to quieten the mind which in turn helps to make you feel relaxed and fall asleep.

Time in bed. Don't spend too much time in bed before you sleep. You don't want to confuse your body and associate work with the same space where you are meant to sleep. When you try to sleep, your body will find it difficult. Instead keep the bedroom for sleeping only. And if you do wake up in the middle of the night and can't get back to sleep, the best thing to do is get up, go to another room and just read for a short while, then go back to bed when you feel really sleepy again.

'Skimping on sleep is not a badge of honour. It will catch up with you sooner or later...'

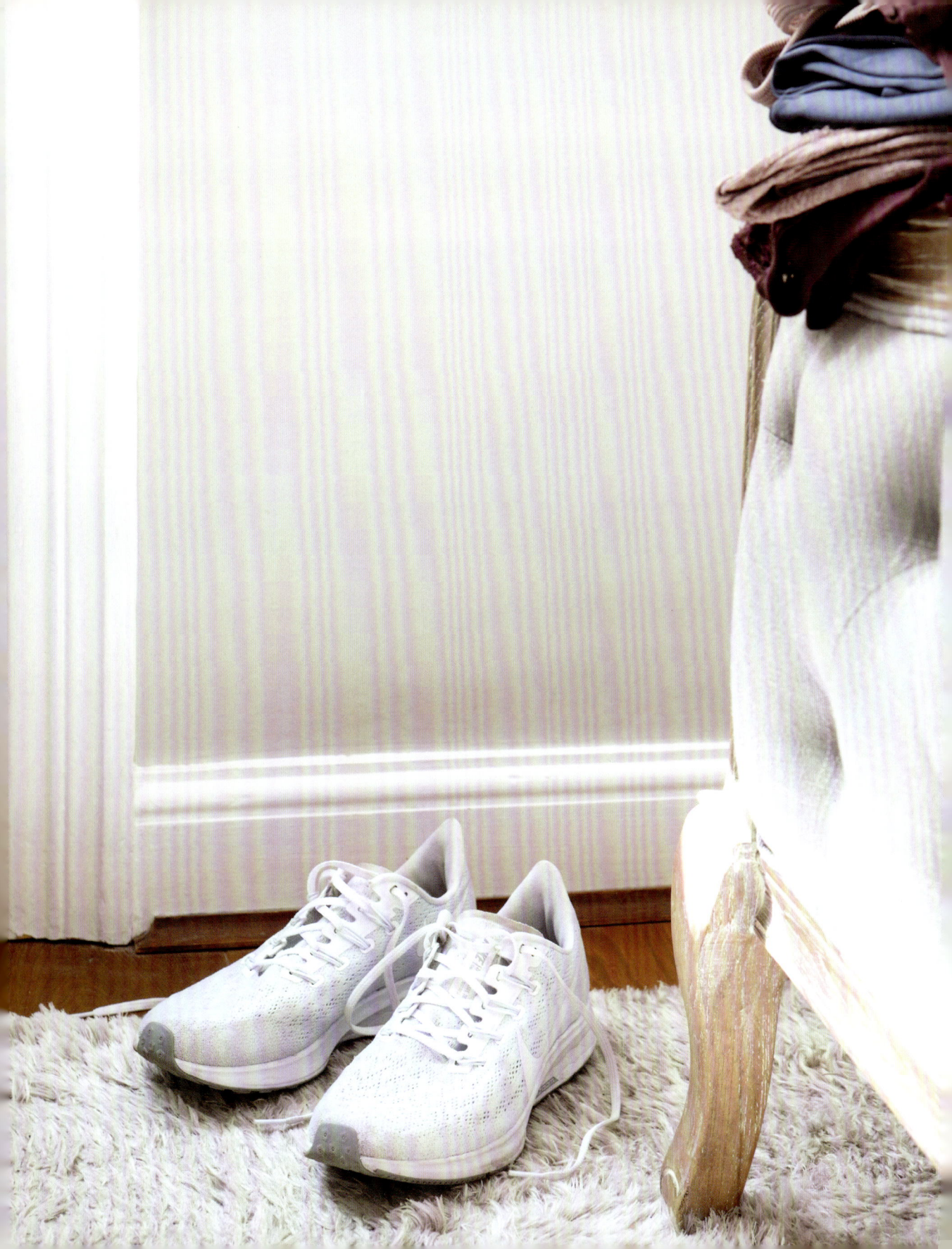

Exercise

Exercise is 1.5 times more effective than antidepressants and therapy. Everyone knows the benefits of exercise and I, for one, am a fan. However, I really believe that we are a nation of overexercisers where people are doing too much. In healthy individuals, exercise gives you energy. But too much exercise can make us tired. Why? Because excessive exercise – particularly the aggressive cardio types such as HIIT (high-intensity interval training), running and boxing – elevates the stress hormone cortisol. In other words, your body mounts a stress response.

If you are fatigued and suffering from burnout, it's really important to not overexercise or overexert yourself. I've had many clients who were working out five or six times a week and experiencing low energy. As soon as we reduced their exercise routine to a more appropriate amount, their energy levels dramatically increased. Remember that exercise is energy out. And if you are fatigued and dragging yourself through the day, a HIIT class straight after work is gonna make you even more tired. When you are fatigued you have to bank as much energy as possible.

TAKE ACTION
Work out how many exercise sessions you are doing each week, then ask yourself if there is something you can cut back on. Can you swap one of your HIIT classes for a yoga class, or just a walk in the park? Make one change this week and monitor your energy to see if it improves.

Undereating

I touched on this in the food chapter, but do you know how many calories you are actually eating in a day? Most people don't. Generally, adult females need 2,000 calories per day and adult males need 2,500 calories per day. I always monitor how many calories my clients eat in one day with either a food diary or an app that can calculate the daily intake.

Many of my clients who come to me with fatigue are actually not eating enough. You have to remember, the food you put in equals energy in. Undereating, coupled with multiple stressors, is a recipe for burnout alone, so skipping meals is definitely to be avoided. The six-week meal plan I have devised for you contains all meals and snacks so you never go hungry or skip meals.

How Can you Measure Your Intake?

My advice is to find out how many calories you actually need.

TAKE ACTION
Do this by visiting a calorie counter website such as MyFitnessPal, and entering details such as your age, height and level of activity. Record how much you are eating daily using a food diary or an app. More sophisticated apps will also tell you the percentage of protein, fats and carbs you are eating.

Difficult Relationships

During my bed-bound days, I was in an unhappy relationship. It was emotionally draining and always sapped my energy. This went on for three years but when the relationship ended my energy improved significantly.

I really believe that you are who you surround yourself with. If you surround yourself with people that make you laugh and lift you and encourage you, it will positively affect the way you feel and the amount of energy you have.

TAKE ACTION
I want you to answer the following questions:

1. Who is draining your energy at the moment?

2. What could you do to surround yourself with people that lift you more?

3. Who would those people be?

4. How can you reach out to them? Would it be a phone call? A coffee? A dinner?

Try to surround yourself with people who have a positive effect. You'll be amazed at the difference this can make to your life.

Social Media

Where do I start? This topic is a minefield and I could write a whole book on it. There are many ways that social media affects our lives and therefore our energy.

We'd all be lying if we said that social media had no control over us whatsoever. And specifically I'm talking about Instagram.

There's a love/hate relationship with these platforms, right? They can be just as toxic as they are amazing. We are all guilty of comparing our lives to everyone else's and also spending waaaaaay too much time on these entertainment apps. But they can consume us and lead to anxiety.

I had a client recently who admitted that scrolling through her Instagram feed left her feeling anxious and affected her sleep.

If social media is causing anxiety then, again, it's causing your body to mount a mini stress response. There is a massive distortion of reality from these apps which can be extremely destructive and stressful.

Most people tend to scroll through their phones at night. This is the absolute worst time to compare our lives with those of others because this is when we feel most tired and vulnerable. So not only are these platforms contributing to anxiety, they are also keeping people awake and affecting their sleep and therefore stress levels and energy.

I think it's crazy that this cycle has become the norm for so many people. Here are my top tips for controlling your social media addiction and stopping scroll overload:

1. Find out how much you're on each app. Your phone should have a function to allow you to do this. It might shock you! You can also check your screen time notification.

2. Put your phone on flight mode from 10pm until 6am every day to help you dim down at night and not get addicted. Sometimes I actually turn off my phone at night and put it in the kitchen drawer so I can completely forget about it. When I do this it instantly makes me feel less anxious and relaxed. I know it sounds scary but it's very liberating.

3. Avoid the search button on Instagram. This is the most dangerous button! It brings up all the people we are likely to compare ourselves with. I avoid this button at all times and it's really helped.

4. Go on a social media detox. Can you come off social media for a few days? I did it for a week and it was much easier than I thought. Do it with a friend or partner to keep yourself accountable. You'd be surprised how refreshing it feels not to be glued to your phone all the time.

5. Schedule in only three specific times each day to check your page – for example, once at 8am, once at 3pm then again at 8pm. That way you are more in control of your phone.

Avoid Comparison

Comparison will kill you. Be you. We are living through a comparison epidemic and it's so unhealthy.

TAKE ACTION
If you are someone who is constantly comparing yourself to other people, then try these ideas:

– Turn off notifications. I'm talking across all apps: Instagram, Facebook, Whatsapp and so on. It's a game changer. Plus it's so nice to not be so distracted all the time.

– Stop following people who don't make you feel good about yourself, or who make you feel anxious when you see them online.

– Get out more. Make plans. Book tickets. Revel in your life OFFLINE more.

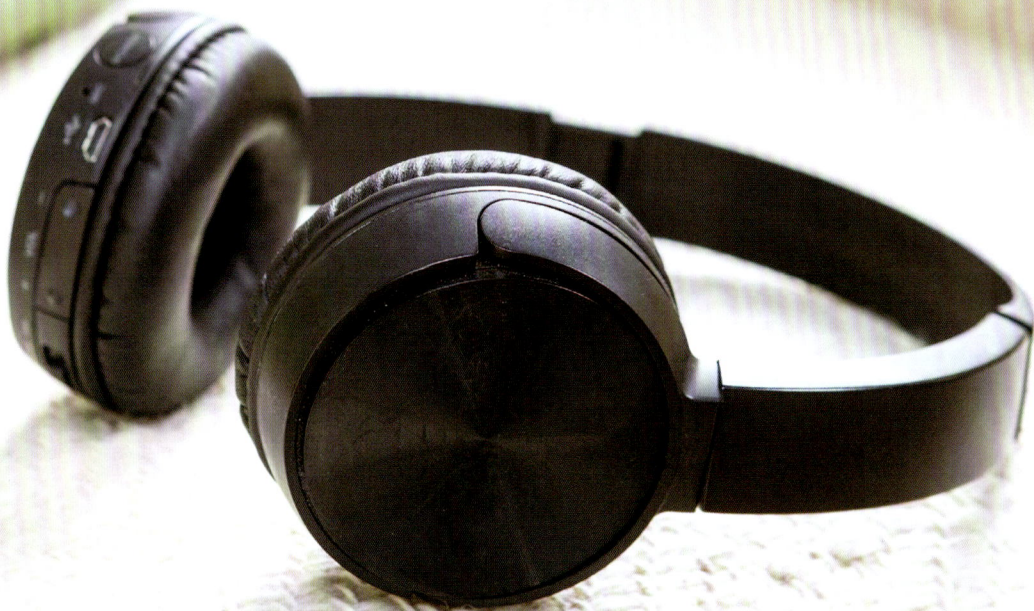

FOMO – Fear of Missing Out

It's crazy that because we are overstimulated, we actually fear that if we are not doing something all the time then we will miss out.

FOMO is most common when we are scrolling through our Instagram feed and watch what our other friends are doing. If we weren't there or didn't get an invite, it makes us feel socially unwelcome and not part of a group or community. This is the kind of anxiety we are experiencing on a daily basis.

TAKE ACTION
Here are some tips to stop FOMO from making you feel rejected:

- Make plans to meet up with friends and family. If you feel like you are missing out, plan your own party. Even if it's a small gathering it will make you feel like the centre of the universe.

- Stay away from social media for a while so you are not constantly looking at what you're missing out on.

- Slow down. Don't rush while you are doing everything. Take time to eat your meals with friends slowly and really be in the moment. Take time to linger over pleasurable experiences rather than rushing through them in the quest for the next thrill.

Create a Support Network

One thing that is critical to recovery is having a strong support network around you. If you do not have this in place, your recovery will be much slower. Don't be afraid to ask for help.

TAKE ACTION
I want you to think about who in your life you can depend on. Is it your partner? Brother or sister? Best friend? Sit down with them and tell them that you are struggling with your energy and finding it hard to cope and need their help for a while. I promise you they will not block this request. The right support network will lend a helping hand.

To Do

This week, please reach out to one person you can ask for help. Perhaps it's to have a lunch and chat about your illness. Or maybe it's to ask them to go food shopping for you or cook a meal or just run errands while you rest and sleep. They don't want to see you like this either. Please remember that there are no medals for pain and suffering. Ask for help.

Happiness

Laughing is good for the soul. Do it loud and do it often. Being happy makes us feel energized. But so many of us are doing things that we hate. A lot of us are in jobs that we can't stand, which leads to feelings of resentment and dissatisfaction. The way we feel can negatively affect our energy levels. If we feel sad or down because we hate the job that we are in, it will sap our energy.

TAKE ACTION

My advice is to identify what it is that you really want in life and write it down. Then I want you to think about what needs to be done in order to get you closer to where you want to be. For example, if you really hate your corporate job and you are passionate about fashion, then what things do you need to do in order to make the move? Do you need to have conversations with friends who work in the industry? Do you need to update your CV or résumé and look for fashion jobs? Do you need to take a short online course to explore the field more? What homework and research can you do in order to be clearer about what it is that you want?

When I was ill in bed I realized that I didn't do ANYTHING that made me happy. I had stopped doing all the things that made me laugh. Eventually I started to watch comedy movies, ask friends to come over for a catch up and a cup of tea, head to a gentle yoga class when I could get out of bed, and spend time with my family. I want you to identify what makes you happy. Do you need to enhance your social life? Do you need to travel more and go on mini adventures? Do you need to spend more time on a hobby?

To Do

1. Write down three things that are sapping your energy right now.

Can you eliminate them from your life?

If not, think about how you can perceive them differently.

2. Write down all of the things that make you happy.

How can you do more of these?

Try to do one thing each week that makes you happy.

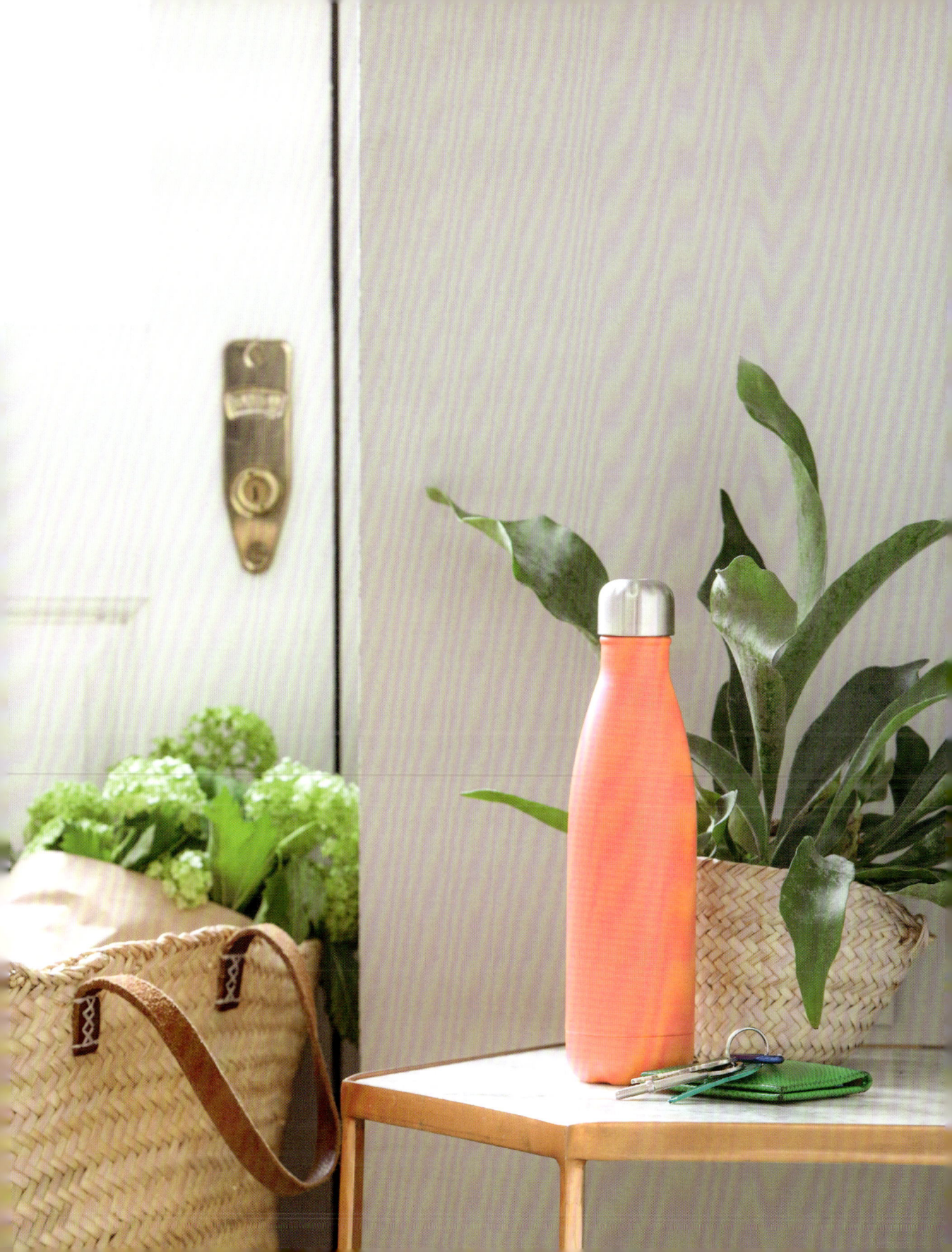

The Traffic Light System

For those of you who are on the floor with your energy and are battling every day with the small things, the Traffic Light System is a great way to gain more control of your energy.

The Traffic Light System is very simple and widely used by doctors with patients who have chronic fatigue syndrome and ME (myalgic encephalomyelitis). To break it down simply, you divide your time into red activities, amber activities and green activities.

TAKE ACTION
It's important to look at your day and identify what type of activities you are doing and where you are spending your energy. If you are extremely exhausted, you need to make sure you are avoiding the red activities and doing more green ones. I call it 'green time'. Make sure you are doing at least one green activity every day, whether it's 30 minutes of yoga, 20 minutes in a warm bath or 10 minutes of deep breathing.

The green activities help to lower cortisol levels and bank energy. I always tell my clients that your body is like a bank account. We need to bank as much money (energy) as possible. If you are constantly in the red, you need to change your activities where you can and start building up some credits. It's so important to be aware of your energy expenditure.

RED ACTIVITIES are the ones that take up a lot of energy and leave you feeling exhausted. These are things like running, aggressive exercise, overworking without sufficient breaks, and all-day events.

AMBER ACTIVITIES are ones that are less strenuous – doing small errands, washing up, cleaning the house, or meeting a friend for breakfast, for example.

GREEN ACTIVITIES are the most important. Examples include gentle yoga, meditation, deep breathing and reading a book. These are the most restorative and help to relax the body and mind.

To Do

1. Think about where you can slow down in your life. Is it at work? Or at home when running your errands? Do you need to delegate more to free up your time? Where can you say no in your life and make yourself the priority?

2. Think about who you can ask for help during this time of fatigue and recovery. What is it that you will ask them to do? The cooking, the cleaning or just listening to your worries?

3. Get more sleep! Put your phone on flight mode. What do you need to do specifically to get more restorative sleep in your life? Do you need to get to bed earlier, drink some reishi tea or take a daily nap?

4. Take a look at your exercise routine. Are you doing too much? Do you need to swap a weekly run for a more gentle walk or yoga class? Think bigger picture here and advise yourself on where to bank more energy.

5. Plan a time in the diary when you and a friend are going to go on a social media detox.

6. Think about where you can add more green time into your diary. Set an alarm to make sure you are doing at least one green thing every day. Is it a walk in the park? A gentle yoga class or just a hot bath?

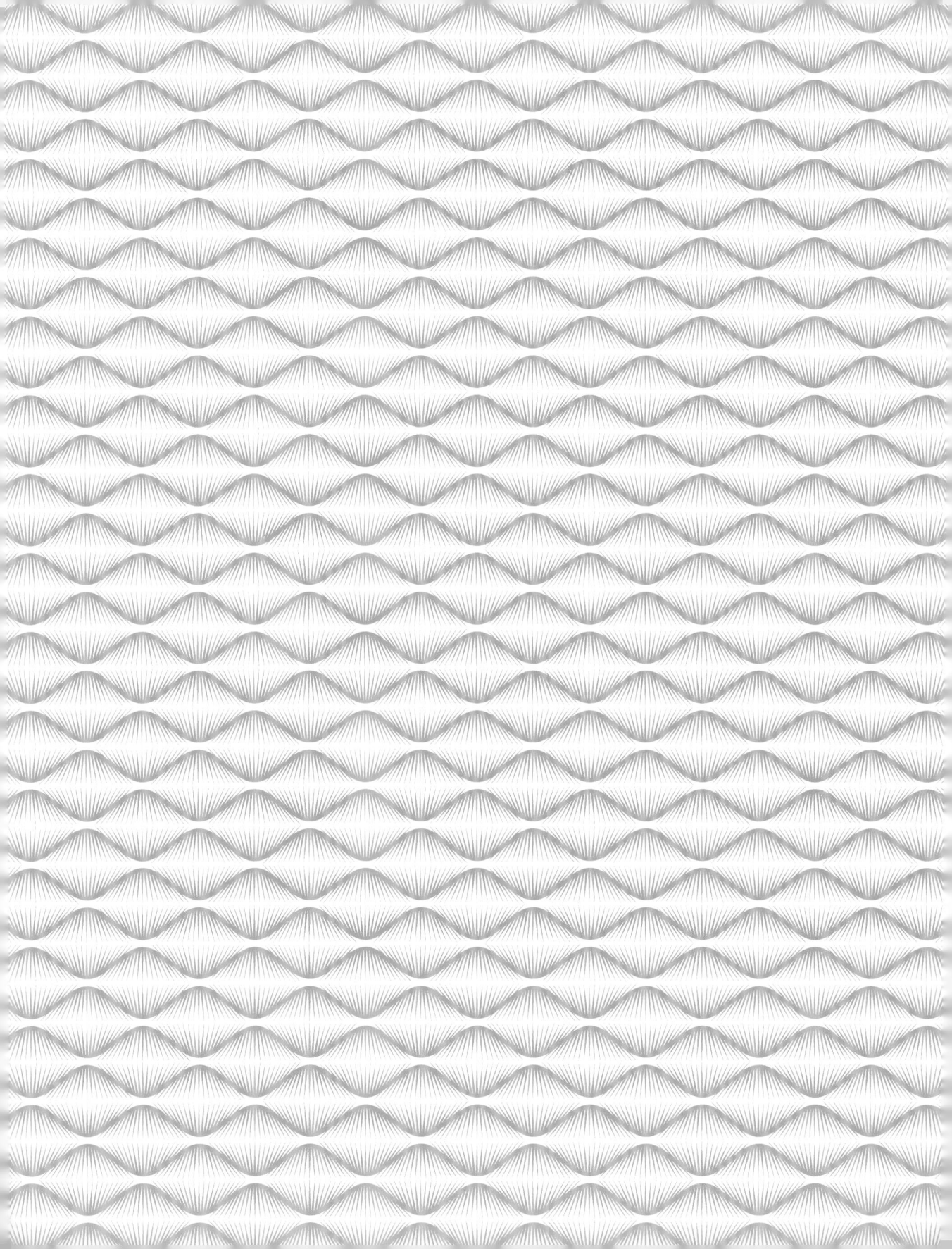

Chapter Six

Navigating Your Mental Health

'There is no health without mental health'

Let's talk about the mental health epidemic we are living in... since Covid we have seen levels of anxiety, depression, ADHD, and suicide rates rise. But why? I believe the key reasons are social media, the effects of the pandemic and a lack of access to care. Our system is broken basically!

We live in a world saturated with comparison, which breeds negative self-talk and self-loathing. And that is a tragedy for our mental health, because a negative mind will never give you a positive life. The average person has 70,000 thoughts per day, and when many of those are negative we are trapped in a continuous loop of toxic thought patterns.

This is why having your own mental health toolkit, which contains everything you need to feel physically and mentally well, is a game changer.

Positive Self-talk

The way you speak to yourself matters the most. But what are you saying? Our inner thoughts can become exhausting. If you are suffering from burnout and constantly thinking you will never recover, then guess what? That's likely to be the case. The most crucial stories are the ones you tell yourself. Your thoughts really do dictate your reality and your inner voice needs to be addressed.

Let's start with this simple fact: by default we usually think negative thoughts. We think more negative thoughts than positive ones.

But negative thoughts limit our daily beliefs. For example, we might think like this...

'I'm never going to get my energy back. I've tried everything and nothing works.'

'I'm never going to be successful. I'm just not cut out for it.'

'I hate my body. I look fat in everything.'

'My boss is awful. She never listens to me, I'm never going to get that promotion.'

Do any of these sound familiar?

When I was bed bound I would always wake up angry that I was not energized and I convinced myself that I would never wake up with energy again. Eventually I realized I needed to re-evaluate my mindset so that it wouldn't sabotage my recovery.

Why? Because your brain doesn't know the difference between real and false, so accepts those negative thoughts as reality. To change your life, you need to change your mindset.

The best way to remove the negative self-talk is to increase the positive self-talk. When we practise acts of self-love we are more positive and secrete more of the happy hormone serotonin. For most of us, praising ourselves doesn't come naturally. But there are no medals for suffering. Having self-love and wanting to be a better version of you is totally acceptable and should be encouraged. Give yourself permission for self-care.

How to Grow Self-Love

TAKE ACTION
1. Stop comparing yourself to others. I know it's hard but it's so destructive. Get into the habit of checking Instagram less frequently or limiting your time on there and put your phone on flight mode for at least eight hours each night. Get some sleep rather than seeing what other people are doing.

2. Do things you love to do. Celebrate who you are and enjoy doing what makes you you. And do it more often. Whether it's cooking, organizing get-togethers, playing sport – do these things because they will make you feel lifted and energized.

3. Identify your value. What is it that you're good at? Recognizing your strengths and writing them down will automatically put you in a self-appreciating state.

4. Exercise and look after your body. If you respect your body you will have more respect for your mind. I don't want you to overexercise because that will exhaust you further, but gentle exercise will catapult you into a happier place of self-love.

5. Acknowledge compliments. I know it's hard but the next time someone gives you a compliment, just say 'Thank you'. Don't demean the gesture. A simple thank you might feel uncomfortable but just allow it to run through you.

'Your thoughts really do dictate your reality and your inner voice needs to be addressed'

Dealing with Negative Thoughts

Did you know that emotional stress has a much greater impact on the adrenal glands than physical stress? If you are constantly worrying about something or having negative thoughts, it is going to make you tired. For this reason it's important to get abreast of your thoughts and not let them get carried away.

TAKE ACTION
Here are some ideas:

1. Write down the thoughts that are going round and round in your head. I want you to be really clear on your thought triggers. Now ask yourself, for each thought, if that negative thought became a reality, what would actually happen? Write the answers to the following questions:

   What's the worst-case scenario?
   What's the best-case scenario?
   What's most likely to actually happen?

   If you do this task you're likely to realize that you'll be able to deal with each outcome, whatever the case.

2. Talk about it. A problem shared is a problem halved. This is often overlooked. Just talking to someone about your worries massively reduces the intensity. It's so powerful. Who can you turn to for help and a chat?

3. Focus on the good. Rather than spending time thinking about what you can't do and don't have, focus on being grateful for the things that you can do and do have. Write in your journal three things that you've achieved each day, however small, and three things you are grateful for in your life. Just thinking about them can improve mood.

   Never underestimate the power of gratitude. It's so easy to take things for granted, especially when you're feeling tired and down in the dumps. But getting real and clarifying what you do have is one of the best things you can do. It will instantly break your existing thought pattern into a more positive one.

4. Next time you have a negative thought in your mind, just ask yourself 'Is that thought useful?' Chances are that nine times out of ten the answer will be a resounding no. Job done.

5. Distract and interrupt. You can interrupt these negative thoughts by doing something else to distract yourself. One of the best ways to do this is to step away from your current situation. So if you are stuck in your head, go for a walk, make a cup of tea or do a gentle workout. It will really shift your perspective instantly.

Dealing with Self-Doubt

We live in a world gripped with self-sabotaging thoughts.

TAKE ACTION
The easiest way to be happy and energized is to manage that doubt. Here's how:

Identify where it's coming from. It's likely that your negative thoughts about yourself are a conditioning. Usually, our way of thinking today stems from events that happened to us in the past and they are still dictating our behaviours. But they shouldn't have a hold any more. Self-doubt occurs because our self-perception is low. It's time to break that pattern of thinking and let it go. To do this, focus on the good and write down everything you have accomplished in the last year. You will be surprised.

A lot of self-doubt comes from fear. Particularly fear of change. But fear shrinks when you walk towards it. It grows when you run away! So having faith and confidence is how you deal with doubt. If you act, doubt becomes minimized. Writing down the worst-case scenario for your worst, most scary problem, and then identifying how you would deal with it is SO effective for minimizing that fear. Especially if it paralyzes you. Try it.

Take a break. Taking time away to shift your focus can really give you a new perspective. Having a break is much needed every once in a while. It can be a real game changer because it interrupts that negative pattern of thinking. When is your next trip away? Can you get out of the city for one day or an evening perhaps? Where have you always wanted to go but never been? What do you need to do in order to make this happen?

Connect with others to get support and reassurance. Sharing your fears and problems with a friend or a loved one always makes them seem less scary and more conquerable. Don't be afraid to reach out and ask for help. Who do you have in your life that you can depend on? Is it time to lean on them a bit more? How about setting up a stronger network of support around you?

The Power of Meditation

Did you know that taking a moment to focus on your breathing is a very simple way of reducing your stress levels? A report published in *JAMA Internal Medicine* found that meditation can help to ease psychological stresses like anxiety, depression and pain. The study found that people who meditated over a short period of time had lower levels of the stress hormone cortisol in the blood stream and lower levels of inflammation in the body too.

So if you are not currently practising mediation, now is the time to start! It was a game changer in my recovery.

TAKE ACTION
I would set two alarms each day to take 10 minutes, do some deep breathing and meditate. You could meditate at 11am or 3pm, or first thing in the morning and before you go to bed – whatever is easiest for you.

Download a meditation app such as Headspace, Calm or Buddhify and use for 10 minutes a day for the next six weeks.

Meditation Exercise

It's important to meditate in a way and at a time that suits you. Sometimes meditation can be in the form of going for a quiet walk or playing an instrument, as long as you start creating time just for you. Here is a simple, but effective, meditation exercise:

1. Sit comfortably on a chair or on the floor. Make sure you will not be interrupted for the next 10 minutes. Close your eyes.

2. Take a deep breath in, followed by a deep breath out.

3. When you are comfortable, at the next inhale touch your index finger to your thumb on both hands and breath out slowly.

4. When you inhale again, touch your middle finger to your thumb, on both hands.

5. Keep repeating this process with all your fingers, until you have inhaled and exhaled 10 times.

6. Once you have completed 10 rounds of breathing, you can go again. Or, when you are ready, open your eyes and slowly get up to continue your day.

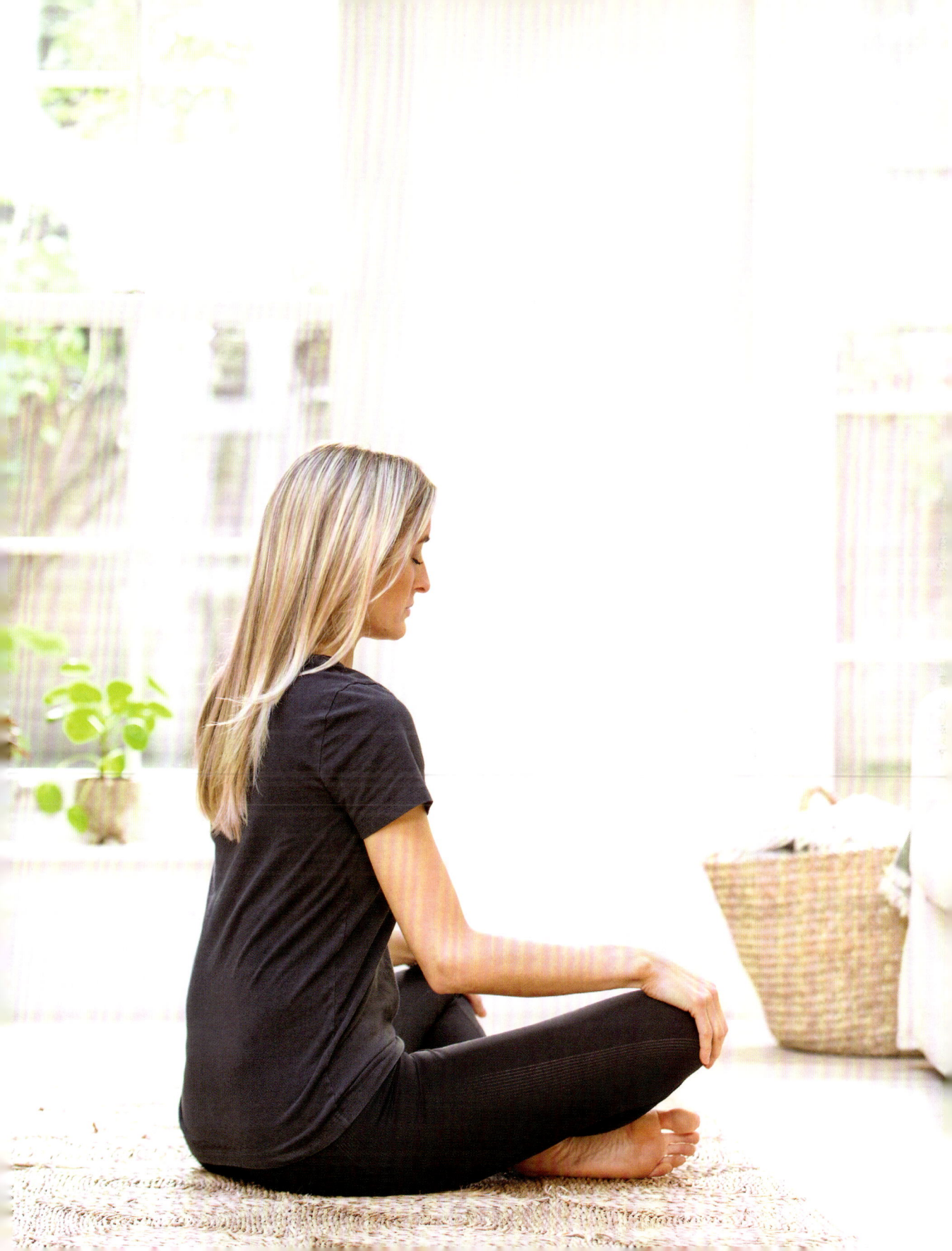

Imposter Syndrome

Chances are you're hearing more and more about imposter syndrome, but what is it? Imposter syndrome, also known as fraud syndrome, is when a person has major doubts about their abilities and accomplishments, despite evidence of competence and success. Instead of thinking how great we are and reminding ourselves of everything we have achieved, instead we think we are just 'winging it' and will eventually be found out and exposed as a fraud.

Sound familiar? Yes, it does to me too. And it's so stupid! But guess what? Everyone suffers from imposter syndrome. Here are some of the typical thoughts you might have when an episode attacks:

'I'm a fake and I'm going to be found out.'

'I haven't got this far on my own, it's mostly down to xxxx.'

'If I can do it, anyone can.'

'What I have achieved is no big deal. I really haven't done anything special.'

'I just got lucky.'

'They're just saying that to be nice.'

Please remember that these negative thoughts are not real. They come from a place of fear and anxiety, they are not based on facts.

Does Imposter Syndrome Sabotage Recovery?

These negative thoughts are emotional triggers which I believe are mini stressors. And we know what emotional stressors do in the body – they trigger the release of cortisol which is not what we want to do while trying to recover from burnout. These negative thoughts are likely to put us in a sad mood and stop us from progressing and moving forward, not just with our recovery, but with our careers and our lives.

I have a confession to make. I still suffer from imposter syndrome from time to time. When people tell me that I'm smashing it or that I'm doing really well, I instantly tell them that I haven't done anything and that it's largely down to the people around me. But that's absurd. Why do we have this built-in destructive mechanism whenever someone praises us or gives us a compliment?

To Do

Instead of feeling like you are inadequate, incompetent and a failure, here are my top tips to get rid of these fraudulent thoughts:

1. Make a list of your strengths and refer back to them when an imposter experience hits.

2. Write down everything you have done and achieved in one week. You will be amazed at how much you have accomplished. It will make you feel instantly satisfied.

3. Find a mentor, or someone you look up to, and speak to them about your insecurities.

4. Get tips from someone who used to be where you are and ask them for advice on how you can grow through this period. Talking with someone who inspires you can also help you see things differently.

5. Decide where in your diary you can schedule in some you time. Use this time to slow down and breathe. This could be meditating with an app, or simply going for a quiet walk in the park.

6. Get out more - take your mind away from your everyday stresses and worries and organize a break away. Can you look at booking a day trip this weekend? Is there an event on soon that you really want to go to? Research something fun and book tickets to enhance the joy in your life and stop you from thinking negatively.

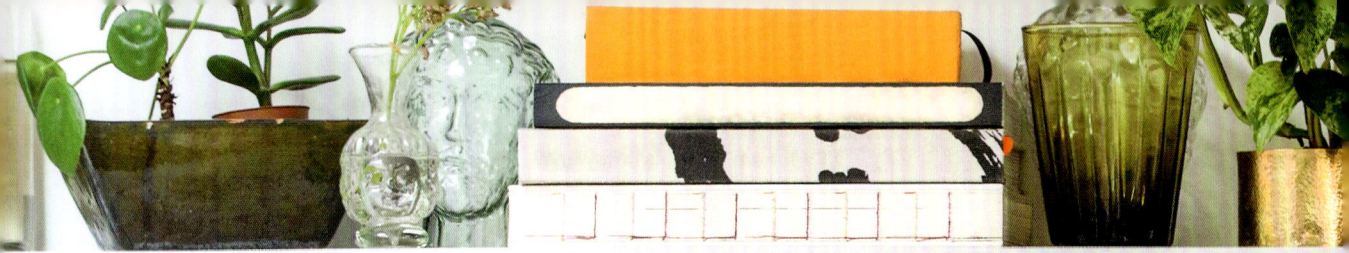

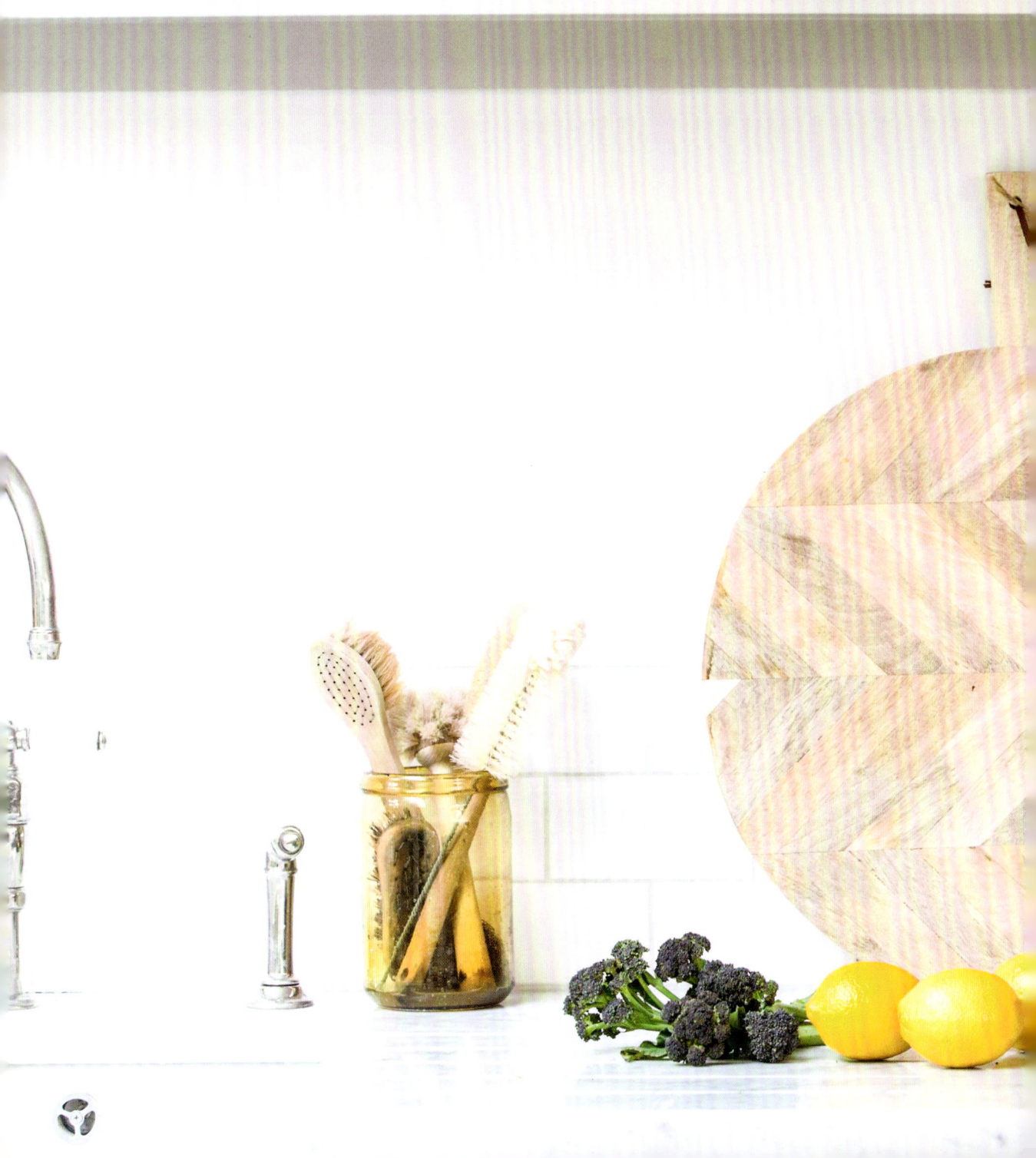

RECIPES

Breakfast & Snacks

Beetroot Smoothie

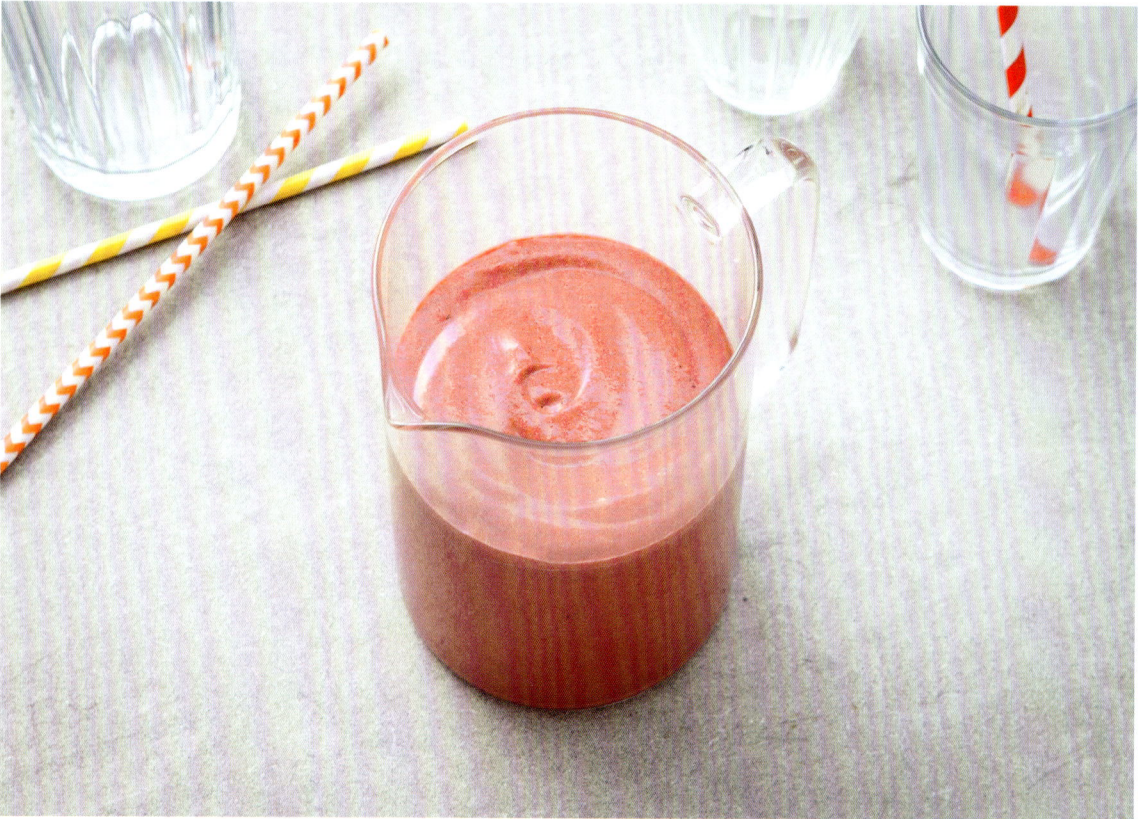

Serves 1

1 banana
½ avocado
1 scoop or 20g (½oz) protein powder
250ml (9fl oz) coconut milk
1 tablespoon beetroot powder
1 tablespoon maca powder

This vibrant smoothie is perfect for post-workout, thanks to its high protein levels. Many brands of protein powder will provide their own scoop, as serving sizes can differ from brand to brand. If no scoop is provided, use 20g (½oz) of protein powder. If you find that you're still hungry after having your smoothie, have one of the snacks from the recipes on pages 126–31.

1. Place all the ingredients in a blender and blitz until smooth.

Chocolate Peanut Smoothie

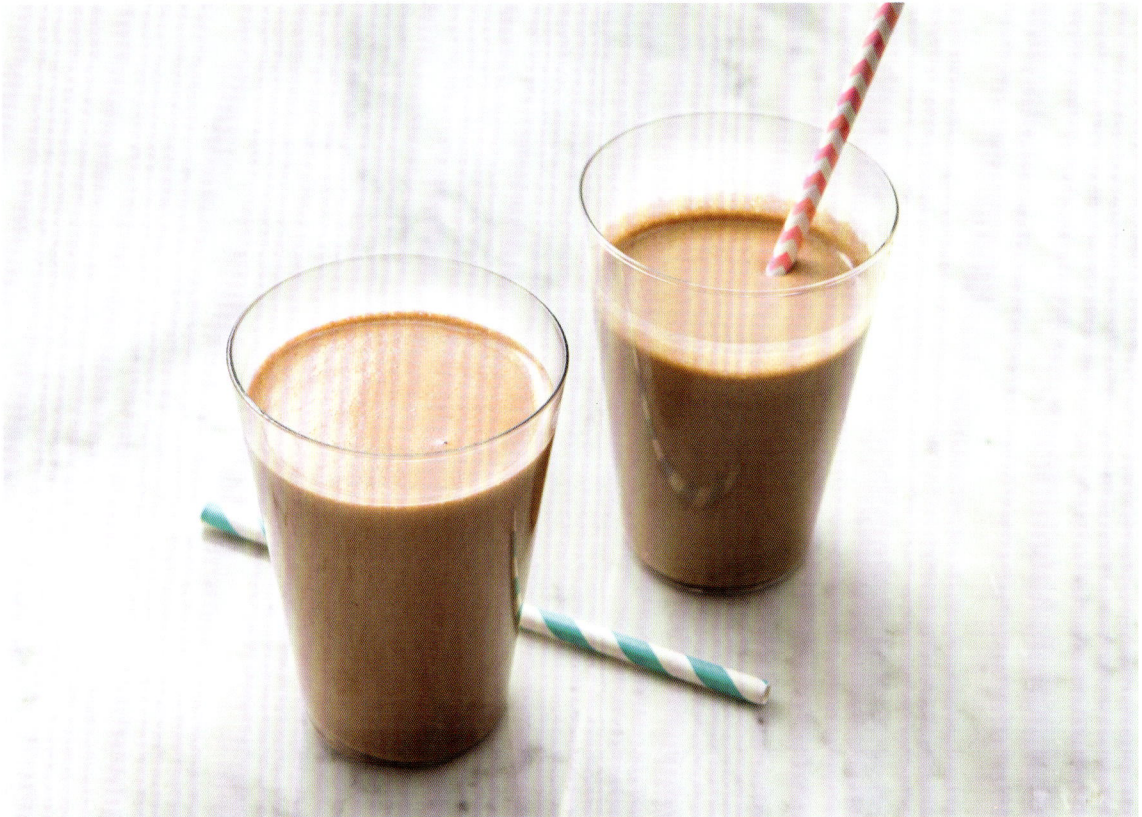

Serves 1

250ml (9fl oz) almond milk
2 tablespoons oats
1 tablespoon cocoa powder
1 scoop or 20g (½oz) vanilla protein
    powder (see opposite)
1 tablespoon peanut butter

This is one of my fave smoothies, because it just tastes so good. Cocoa powder contains an amino acid called tryptophan, which gets converted to serotonin – the happy hormone – in the body. So not only does this smoothie taste good, it makes you feel good too! If you find that you're still hungry after having your smoothie, have one of the snacks from the recipes on pages 126–31.

1. Place all the ingredients in a blender and blitz until smooth.

Fresh Mint Smoothie

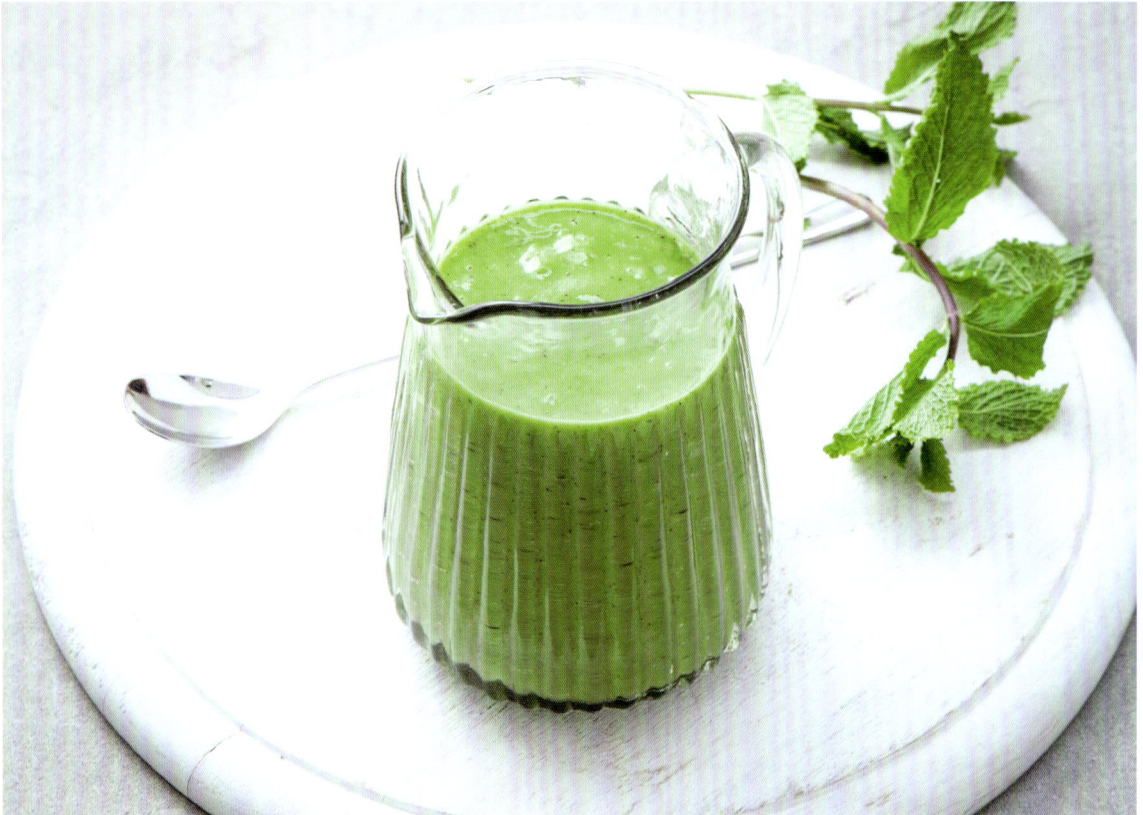

1 banana
1 kiwi
½ avocado
handful of spinach
1 mint sprig
250ml (9fl oz) coconut water

Mint is one of my favourite herbs. It's excellent for soothing the gut and for digestive health in general. If you have any digestive complaints, this is the smoothie for you. If you find that you're still hungry after having your smoothie, have one of the snacks from the recipes on pages 126–31.

1. Place all the ingredients in a blender and blitz until smooth.

Chocolate Protein Smoothie

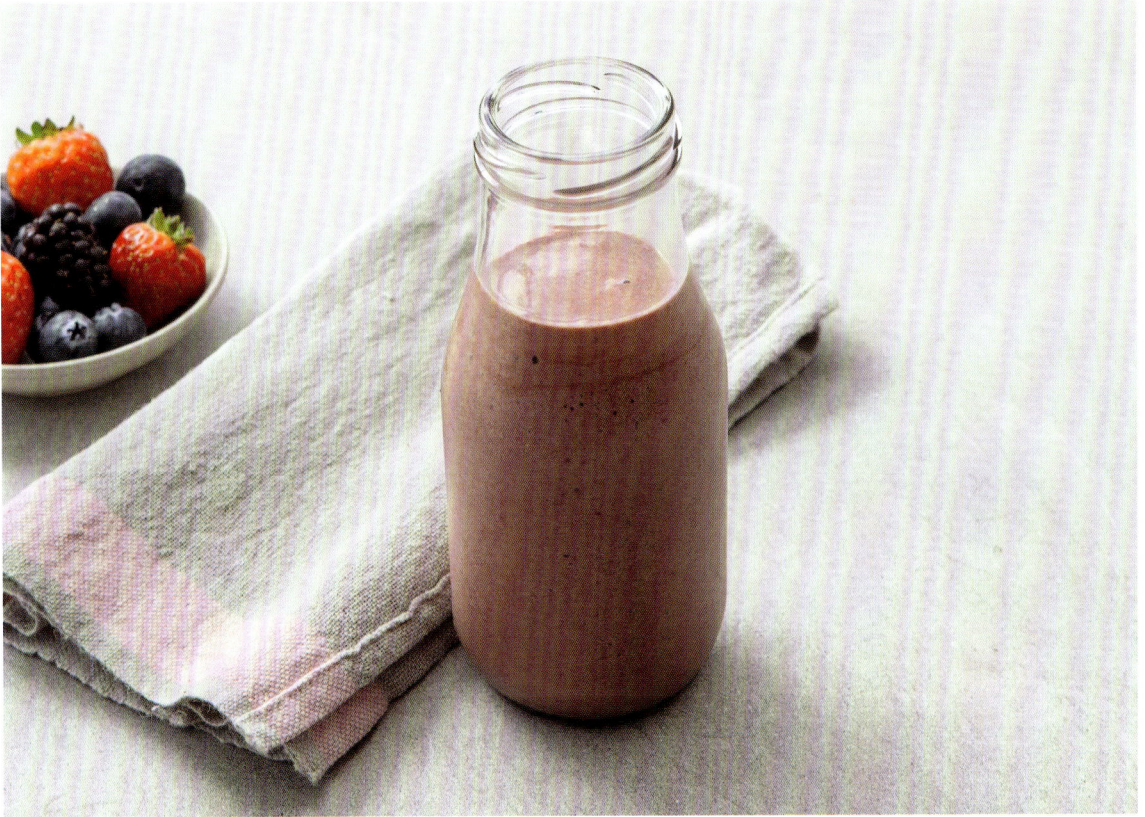

1 banana
handful of frozen berries
1 tablespoon cocoa powder
250ml (9fl oz) almond milk
1 scoop or 20g (½oz) protein powder
  (see page 104)

Remember, if you suffer with digestive complaints, use a dairy-free rice protein powder, as they are easier to digest than other protein powders. If you find that you're still hungry after having your smoothie, have one of the snacks from the recipes on pages 126–31.

1. Place all the ingredients in a blender and blitz until smooth.

Mango, Strawberry & Coconut Smoothie

Strawberries – who doesn't like them? They are packed with vitamin C antioxidants. They are nutrient-dense and a good source of potassium (which makes us feel energized and uplifted). If you find that you're still hungry after having your smoothie, have one of the snacks from the recipes on pages 126–31.

Serves 1

1 mango, pitted and chopped
handful of strawberries
125ml (4fl oz) coconut milk
125ml (4fl oz) water

1. Place all the ingredients in a blender and blitz until smooth.

SHOPPING TIP

When you walk into any supermarket,
generally ALL of the healthy foods
are on the OUTSIDE AISLES, while all
of the refined and processed foods are
in the middle.

SO LIVE ON THE EDGE! Make sure you
spend most of your time in the fresh
produce section.

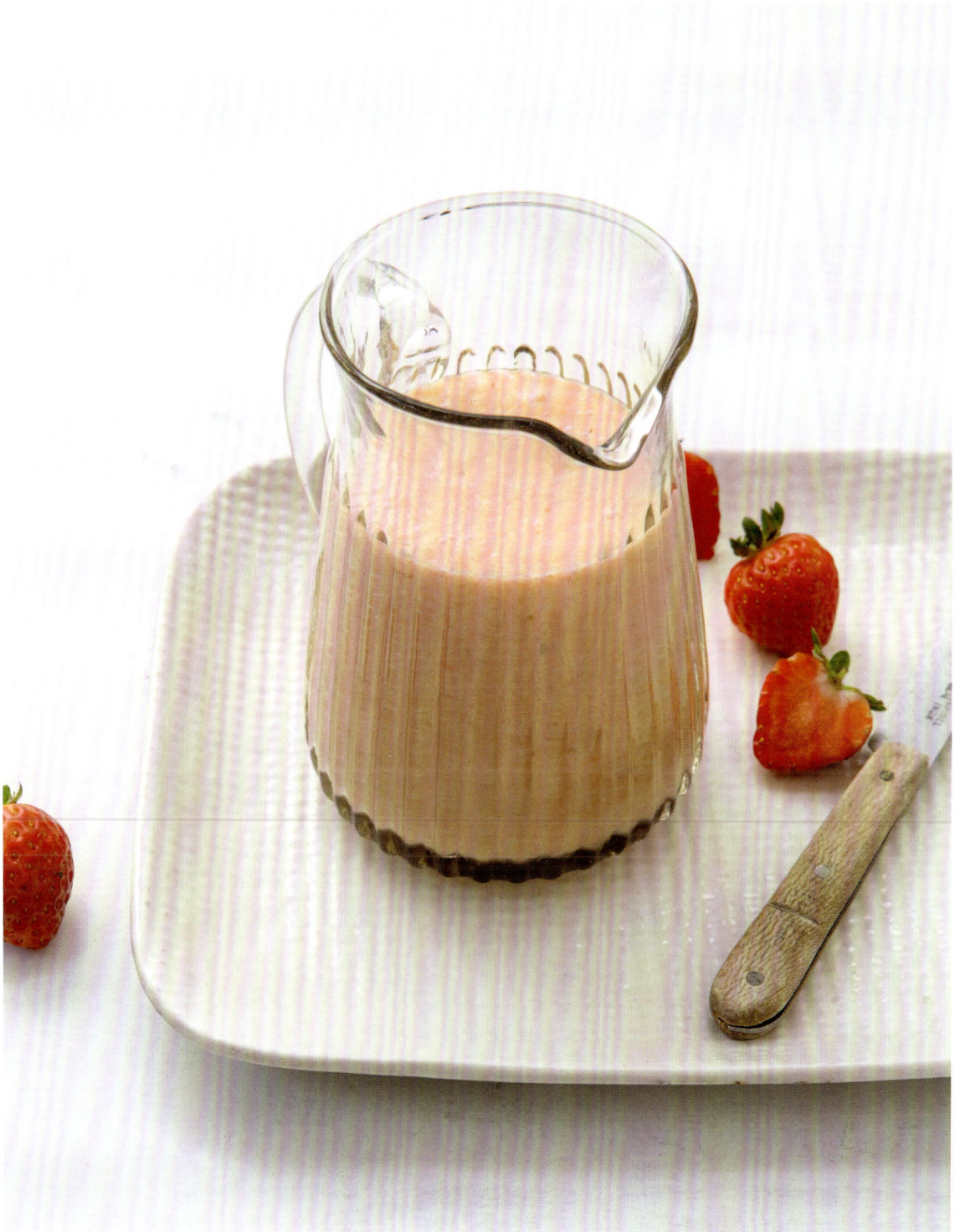

Sunshine Smoothie

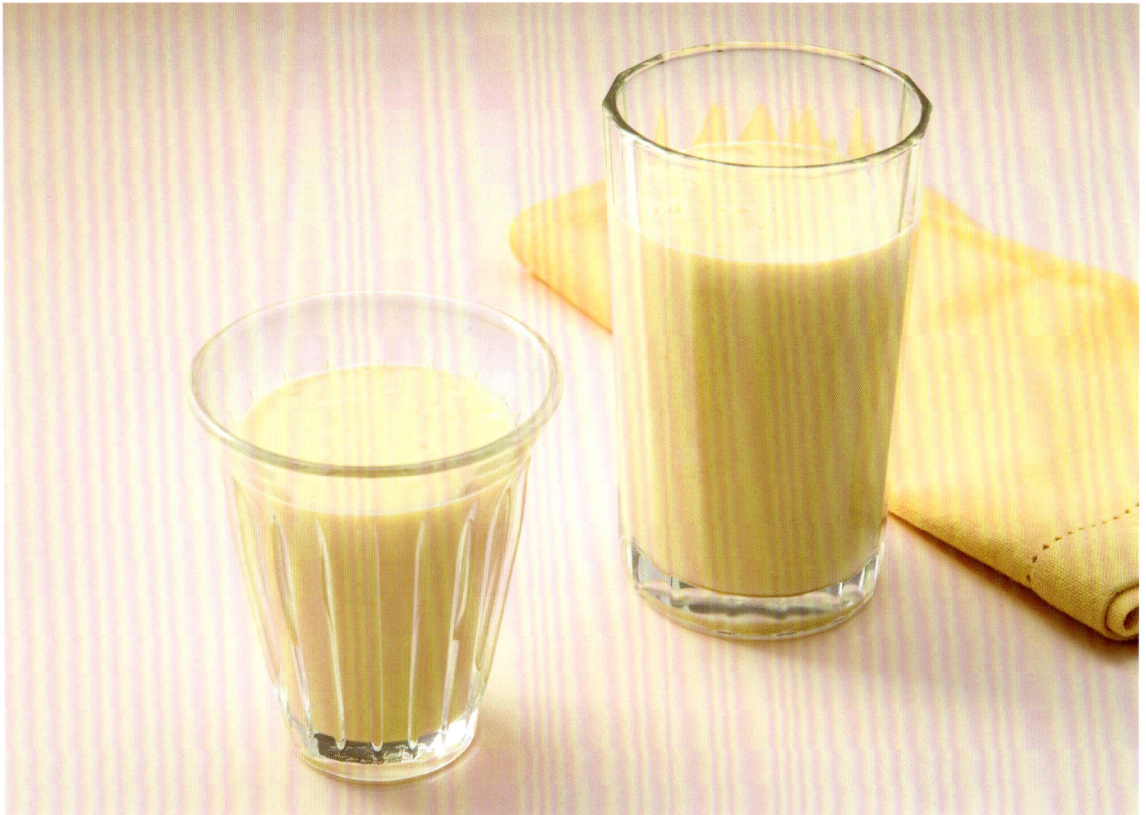

1 mango, pitted and chopped
250ml (9fl oz) unsweetened
   soya yogurt
splash of coconut or almond milk

This smoothie is quite literally sunshine in a glass. Mango is packed with vitamin C and vitamin A, which are both excellent for the skin. Soya yogurt is a great source of protein and phytonutrients (nutrients found in plants). If you find that you're still hungry after having your smoothie, have one of the snacks from the recipes on pages 126–31.

1. Place all the ingredients in a blender and blitz until smooth.

Blueberry Smoothie

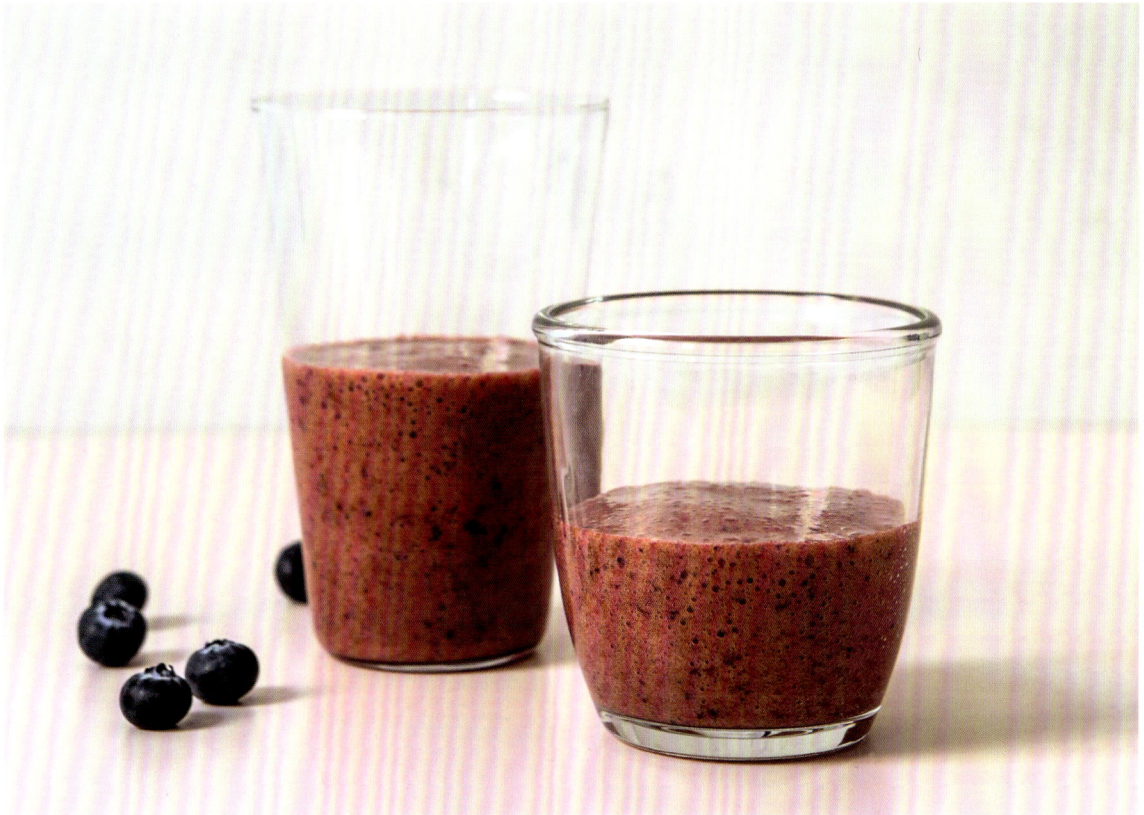

100g (3½oz) blueberries
large handful of blackberries
1 scoop or 20g (½oz) berry or vanilla
    protein powder (see page 104)
250ml (9fl oz) coconut water

Blueberries are the kings of antioxidants. They are high in the mineral manganese, which helps convert fats, proteins and carbohydrates into energy. If you find that you're still hungry after having your smoothie, have one of the snacks from the recipes on pages 126–31.

1. Place all the ingredients in a blender and blitz until smooth.

Pina Colada Smoothie

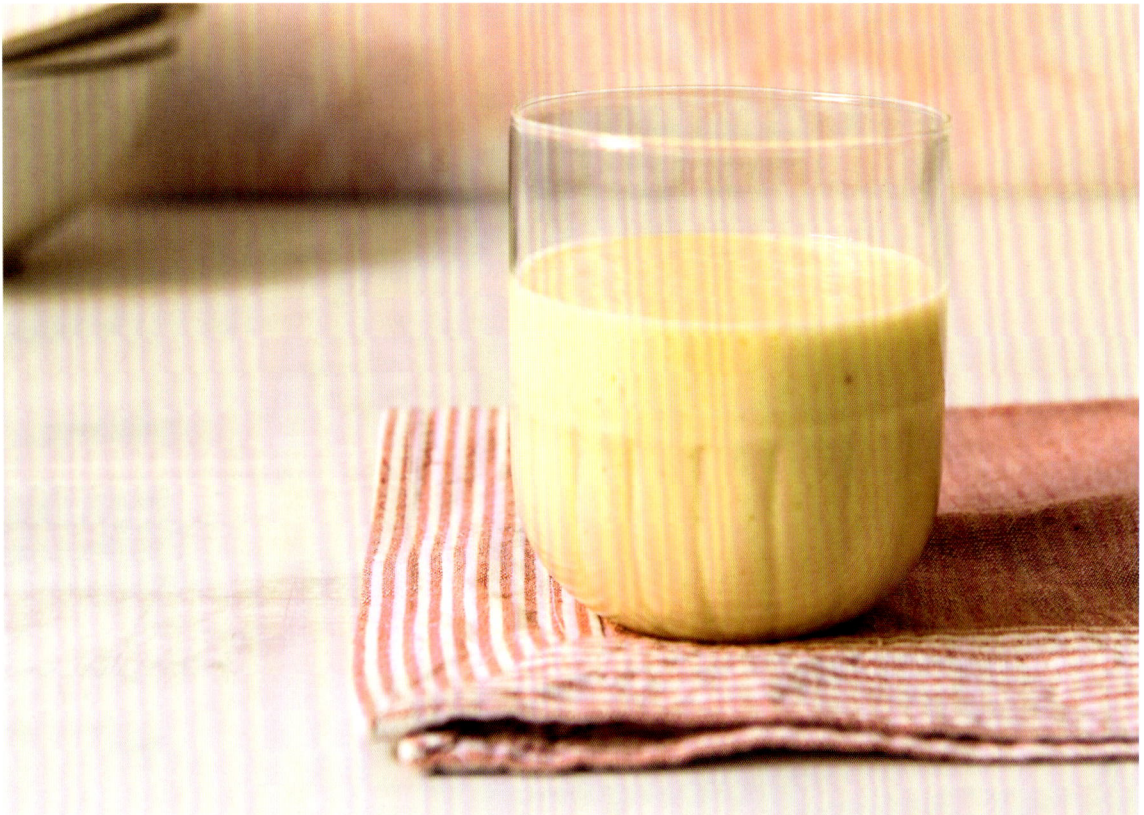

Serves 1

200g (7oz) chopped fresh pineapple
250ml (9fl oz) coconut milk
1 scoop or 20g (½oz) vanilla whey
protein powder (see page 104)

Fresh pineapple contains an enzyme called bromelain. Bromelain has anti-inflammatory properties and can help with digestion. If you find that you're still hungry after having your smoothie, have one of the snacks from the recipes on pages 126–31.

1. Place all the ingredients in a blender and blitz until smooth.

Blue Spirulina Smoothie

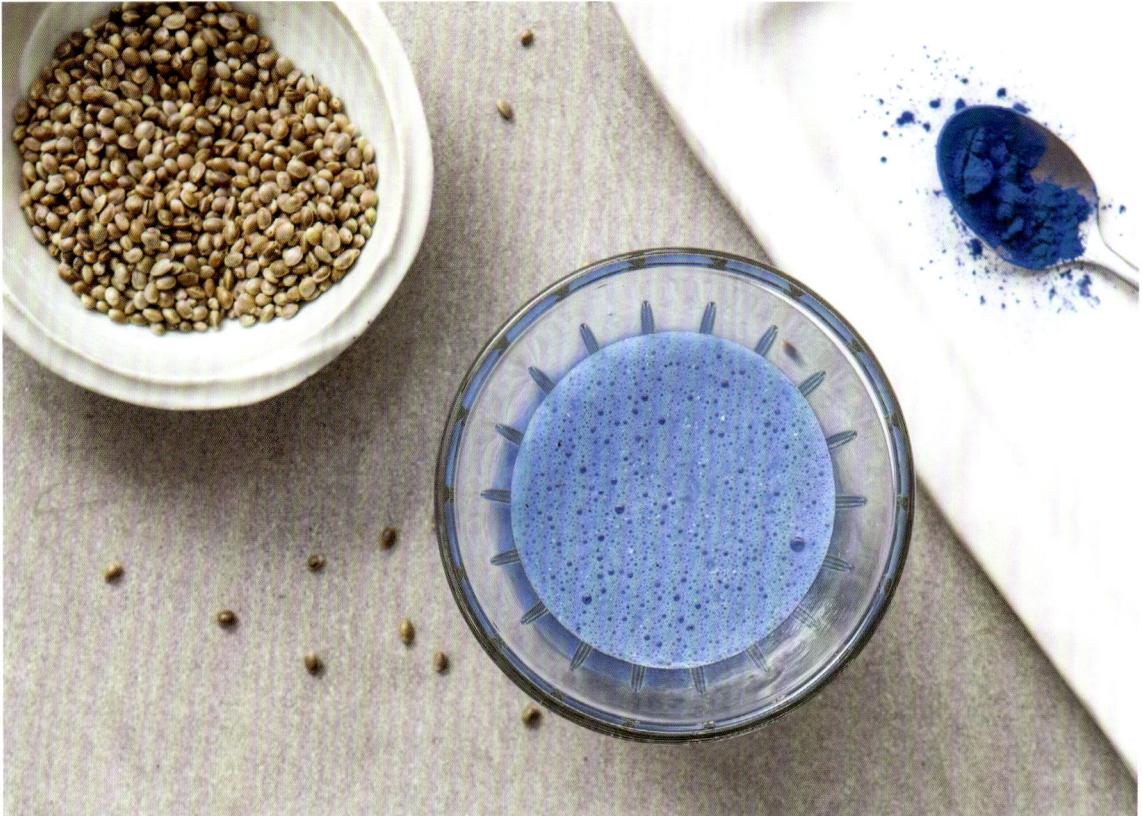

Serves 1

1 teaspoon blue spirulina powder
250ml (9fl oz) coconut water
1 scoop or 20g (½oz) whey protein
    powder (see page 104)
1 frozen banana
handful of hemp seeds
3 tablespoons yogurt

Blue spirulina is a an algae which grows in ponds and lakes. It is rich in protein, iron, sodium and magnesium. In fact, it is a powerhouse of nutrients. The fabulous colour comes from the protein phycocyanin. I prefer it to normal spirulina because it doesn't have that fishy taste. If you find that you're still hungry after having your smoothie, have one of the snacks from the recipes on pages 126–31.

1. Place all the ingredients in a blender and blitz until smooth.

Raspberry Coconut Smoothie

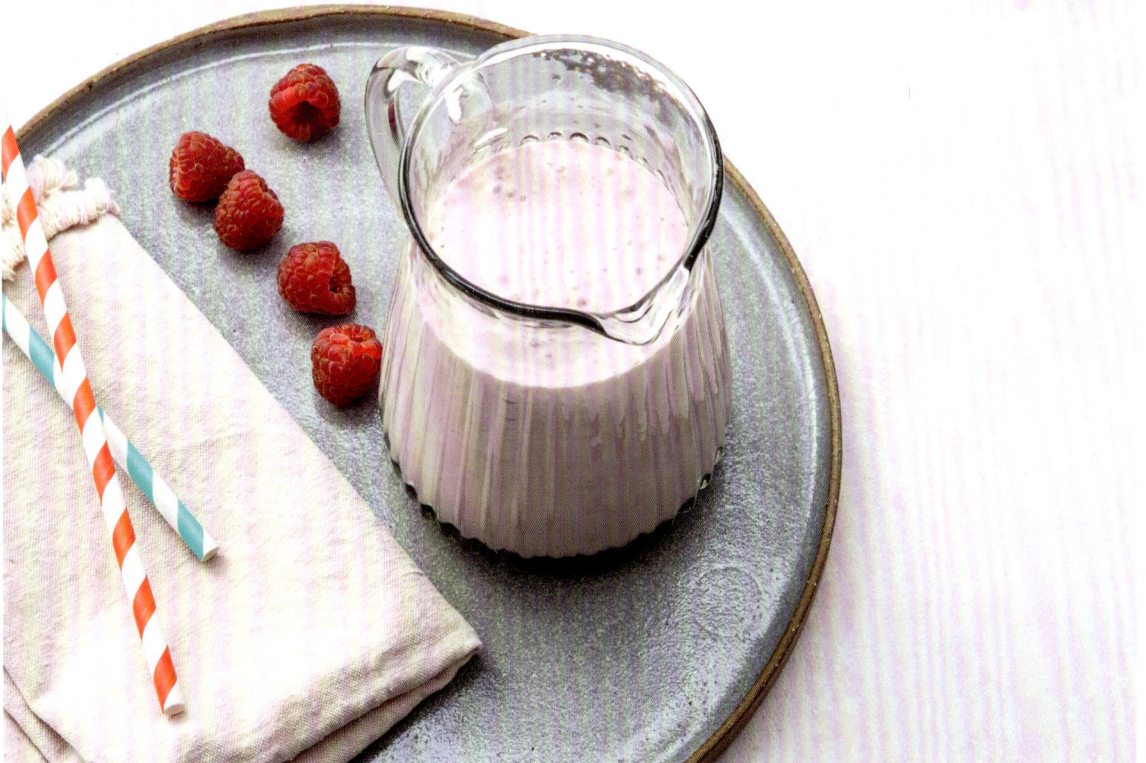

Serves 1

125g (4½oz) frozen raspberries
250ml (9fl oz) coconut milk
4 heaped tablespoons soya yogurt
1 scoop or 20g (½oz) vanilla whey
    protein powder (see page 104)

Did you know that there are more than two hundred types of raspberries and that each raspberry contains an average of a hundred seeds? Raspberry seeds are packed with antioxidants and vitamin C, and are a good source of fibre. If you find that you're still hungry after having your smoothie, have one of the snacks from the recipes on pages 126–31.

1. Place all the ingredients in a blender and blitz until smooth.

Vanilla Protein Smoothie

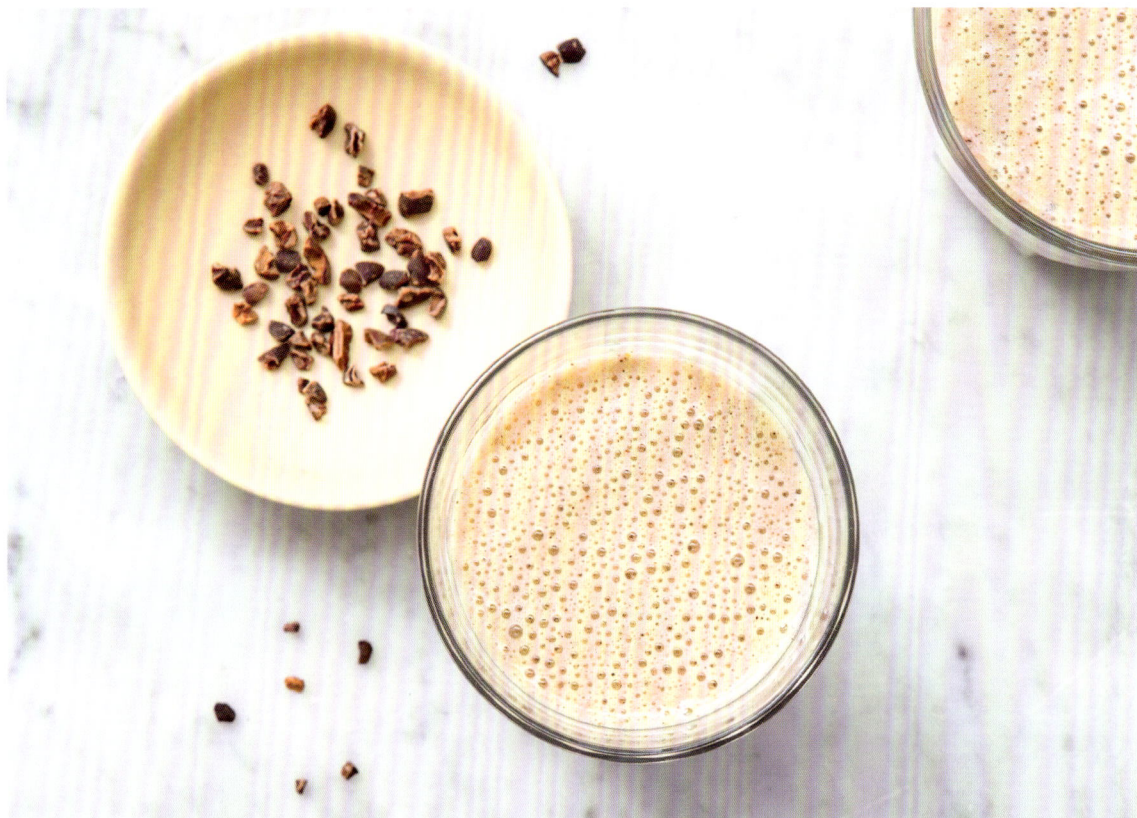

Serves 1

1 banana
2 medjool dates, pitted
250ml (9fl oz) almond milk
1 scoop or 20g (½oz) vanilla protein
   powder (see page 104)
1 tablespoon cacao nibs

I've used two medjool dates in this smoothie as they are excellent sources of fibre, iron, magnesium and potassium. If you find that you're still hungry after having your smoothie, have one of the snacks from the recipes on pages 126–31.

1. Place all the ingredients in a blender and blitz until smooth.

Power Smoothie

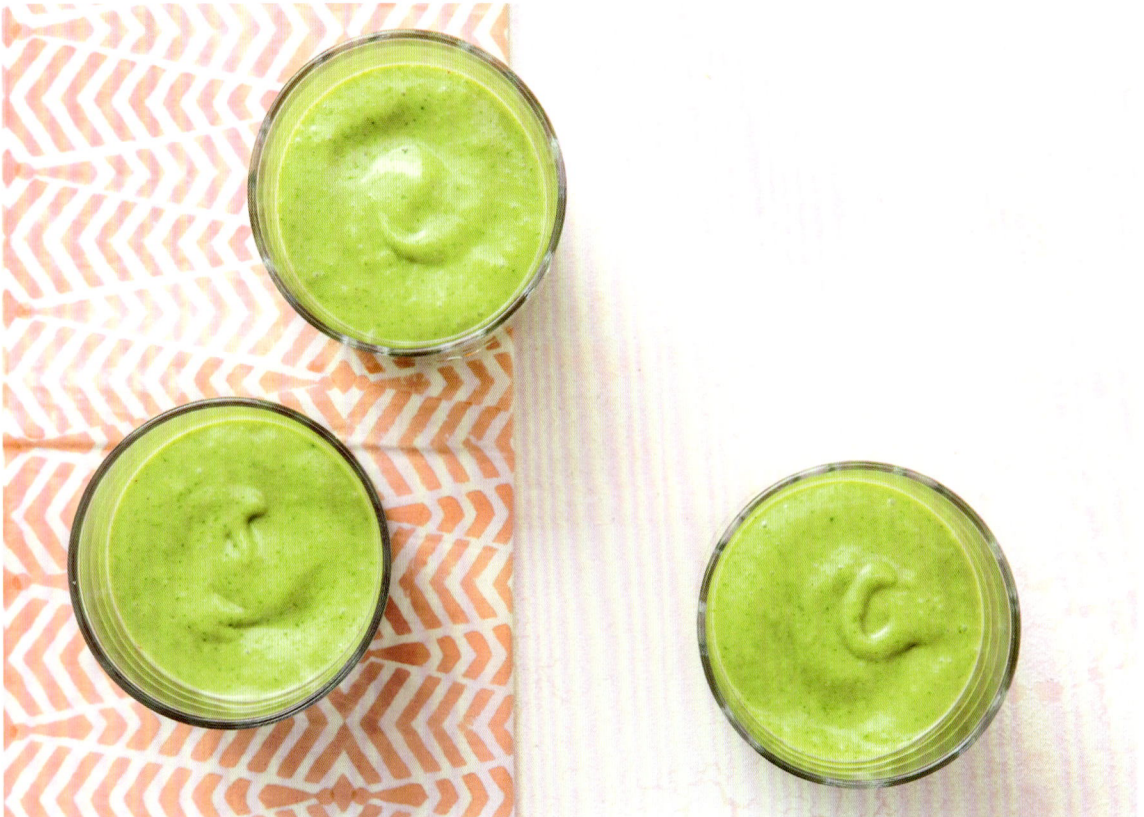

½ avocado
1 banana
handful of spinach
1 scoop or 20g (½oz) protein powder
   (see page 104)
½ teaspoon matcha powder
250ml (9fl oz) coconut milk
1 teaspoon coconut oil

Matcha powder is packed with antioxidants and amino acids. While it does contain a small amount of caffeine (roughly 30mg per cup), the amino acid L-theanine found in matcha actually helps to prevent the energy crash that caffeine usually causes. If you find that you're still hungry after having your smoothie, have one of the snacks from the recipes on pages 126–31.

1. Place all the ingredients in a blender and blitz until smooth.

Fruity Quinoa Bowl

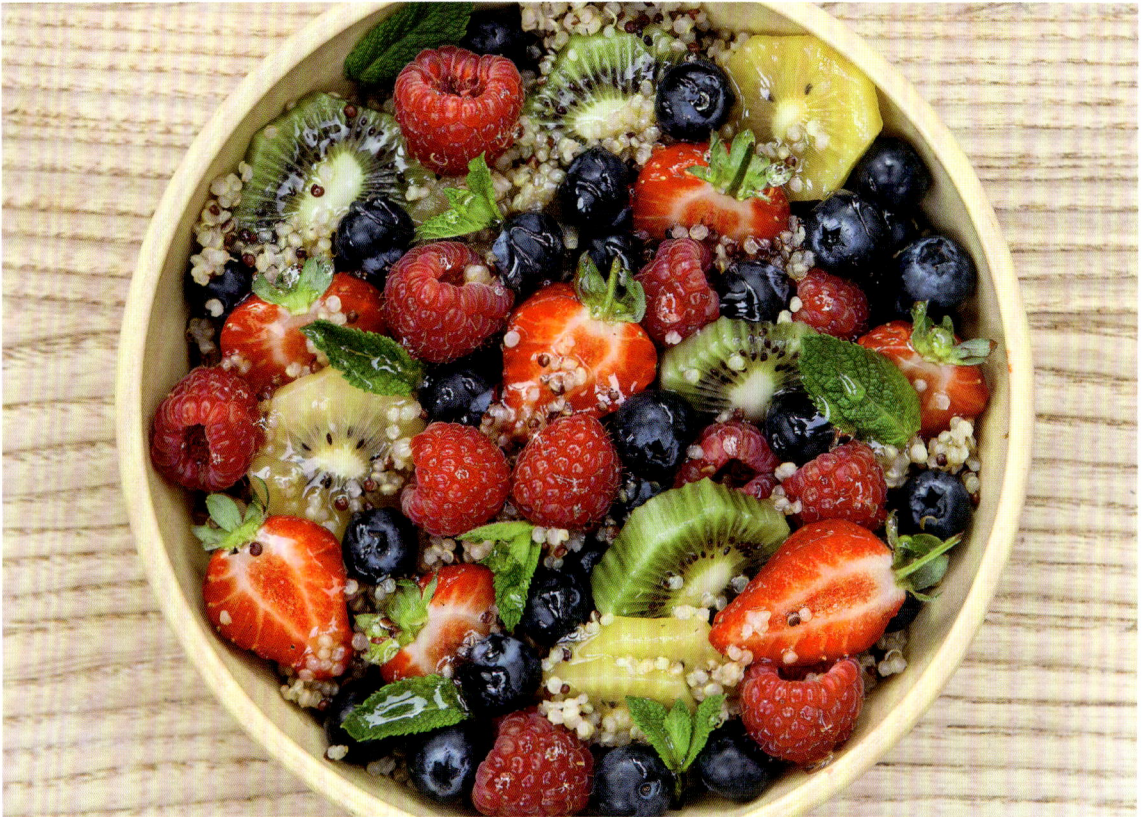

<u>Serves 1</u>

100g (3½oz) quinoa
250ml (9fl oz) water

To serve:
berries, banana or kiwi
chopped roasted almonds
lemon or lime juice
runny honey, for drizzling

As quinoa contains all of the nine essential amino acids (see page 56), it is one of the best plant-based sources of protein. It is also a great source of fibre, magnesium, B vitamins, iron and potassium, all of which have a role to play in providing energy to the body.

1. Place the quinoa and measured water in a saucepan over a medium heat. Bring to the boil, reduce the heat and cook for about 15 minutes, or until tender. Drain through a sieve and set aside for 15 minutes to cool.

2. Place the quinoa in a bowl and toss with fresh berries, slices of banana or kiwi and some roasted almonds. Squeeze over a little lemon or lime juice and a drizzle of runny honey.

Banana & Mixed Berry Pancakes

Bananas are an excellent source of potassium, which is required to keep blood pressure levels healthy. They are also excellent sources of B6 and contain good amounts of fibre.

Serves 2

2 eggs, beaten
4 tablespoons oatmeal or
    almond flour
1 teaspoon baking powder
olive oil, for greasing

To serve:
1 banana, thinly sliced
handful of mixed berries
honey, for drizzling
sesame seeds, for sprinkling

1. Beat the eggs in a jug. Add the oatmeal and baking powder and stir to form a smooth batter.

2. Place a shallow frying pan over a medium heat and grease the pan with a little olive oil on a piece of kitchen paper. When the pan is hot, spoon 2–3 tablespoons of batter into the pan to make each pancake, cooking them 2 at a time – any more will make it difficult to flip them.

3. Cook for about 4 minutes on each side until golden brown, greasing the pan again before each new batch. Serve with sliced bananas, berries, a drizzle of honey and a sprinkling of sesame seeds.

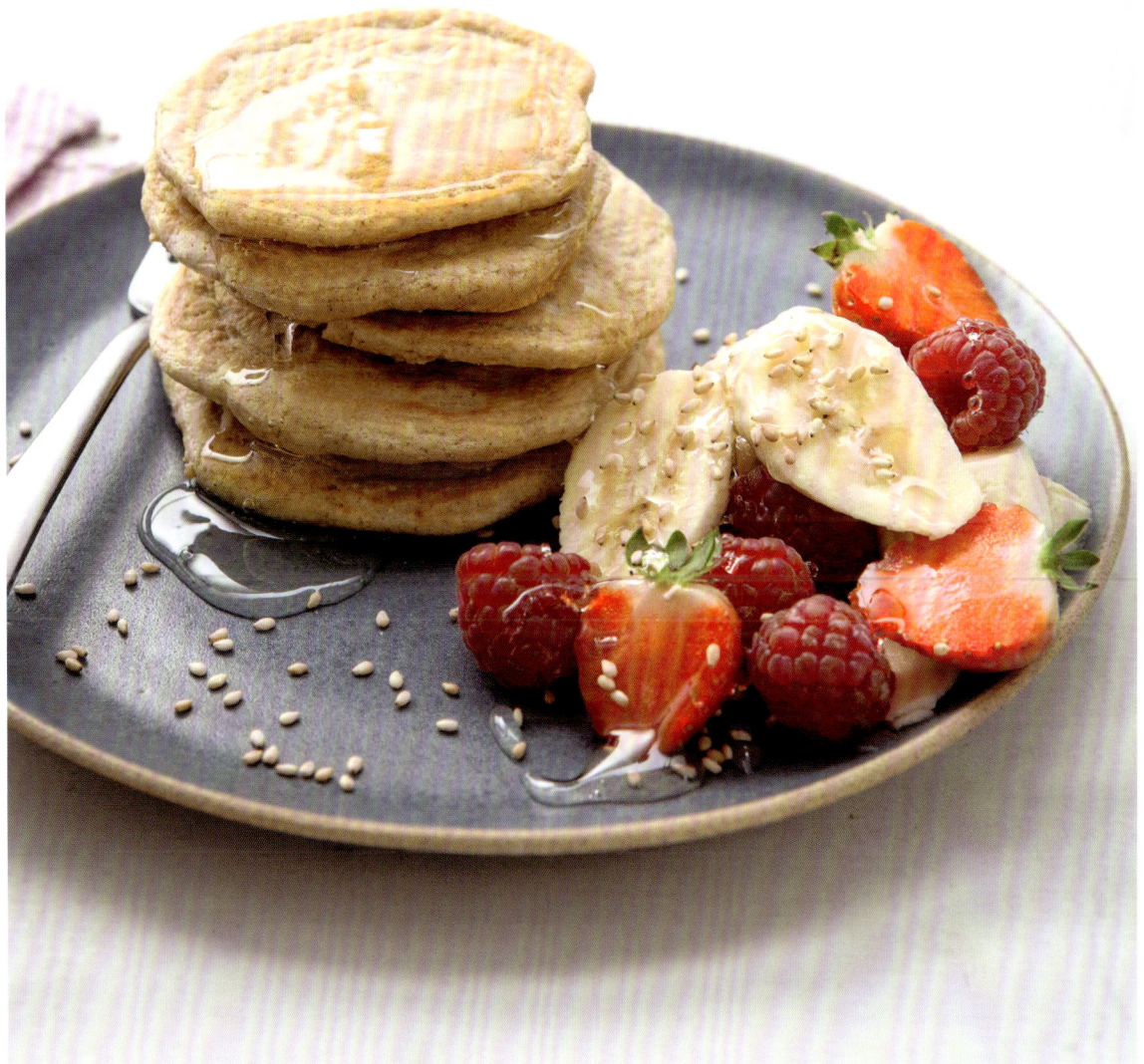

Poached Eggs on Veggies

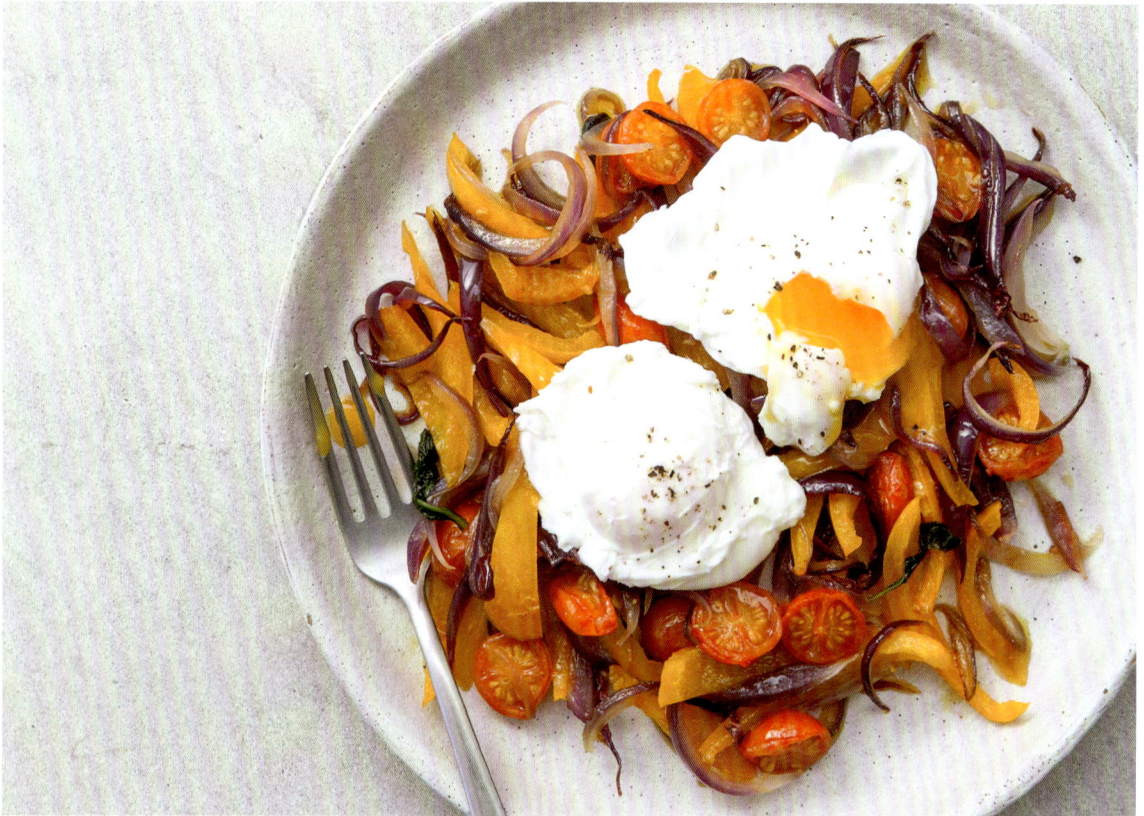

Serves 1

1 tablespoon olive oil
1 red onion, sliced
1 red or yellow pepper, cored,
   deseeded and sliced
handful of cherry tomatoes, halved
3 basil leaves, torn
splash of white wine vinegar
2 eggs
salt and black pepper

Two eggs will give you roughly 15g (½oz) of protein, so this dish is an excellent start to the day.

1. Heat the olive oil in a frying pan over a medium heat and add the onion and red or yellow pepper. Cook, stirring often, for 6–7 minutes, or until the vegetables are tender. Season to taste, add the tomatoes and basil and cook for a further 2–3 minutes to soften the tomatoes.

2. Meanwhile, bring a small saucepan of water to the boil. Add a pinch of salt and a splash of white wine vinegar. Reduce the heat to a very gentle simmer and carefully break the eggs, one at a time, into the pan, spacing them well apart. Remove the pan from the heat, cover and leave for 5–6 minutes, or until the eggs are cooked to your liking.

3. Place the veggies on a plate and top with the eggs.

Black Beans & Avocado on Toast

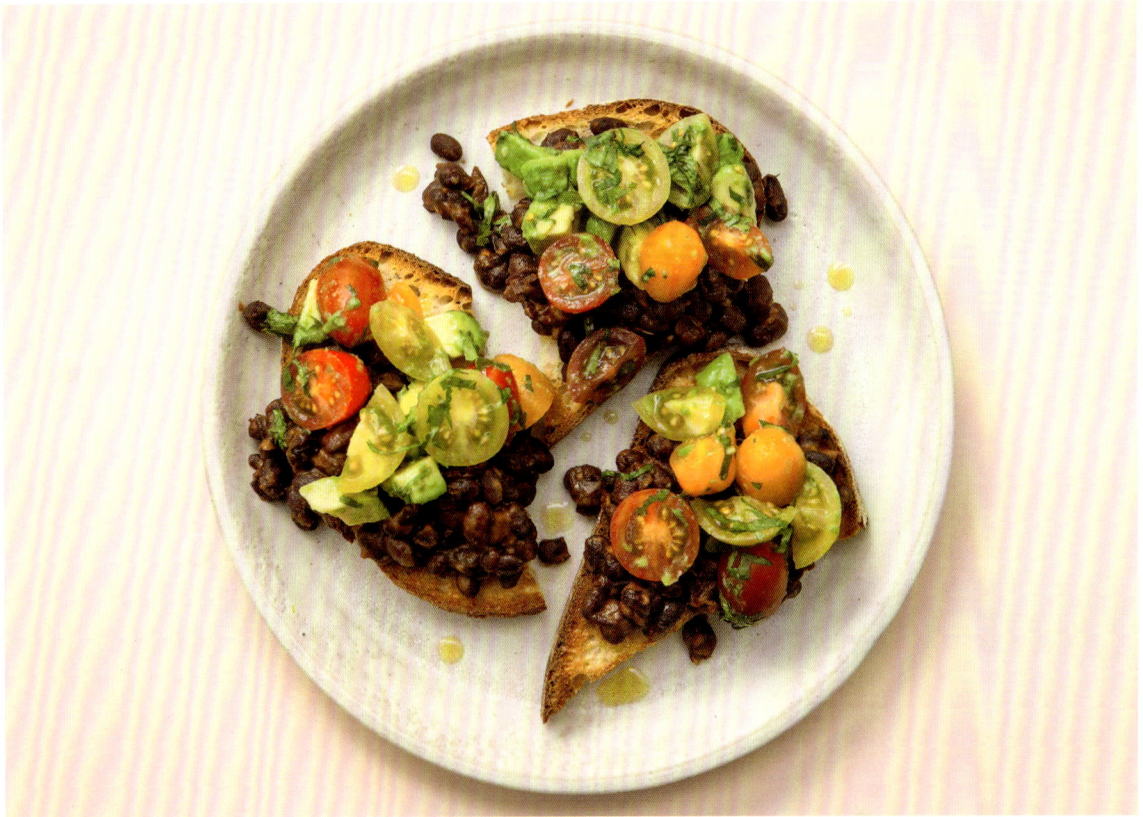

Serves 1

1 tablespoon olive oil

400g (14oz) can black beans, rinsed and drained

2 garlic cloves, crushed

½ teaspoon paprika

juice of 1 lime

½ avocado, chopped

handful of cherry tomatoes, halved

handful of chopped coriander

salt and black pepper

gluten-free toast, to serve

Ever heard the expression 'to be full of beans'? Because of their high vitamin B content, beans literally give you energy. Black beans contain high amounts of B1 and folate, which are co-factors for producing ATP in the body (your body's energy molecule). They are also a good source of iron and magnesium.

1. Heat the olive oil in a small saucepan over a medium heat and add the beans. Stir in the garlic, paprika and lime juice, season to taste and cook for 5–10 minutes, or until the beans start to soften.

2. Meanwhile, mix the avocado, tomatoes and coriander together and season lightly.

3. Serve the beans on gluten-free toast with the avocado mixture on top.

Beetroot Hash with Eggs

I'm a big fan of beetroot, not only because of its energy-giving properties, but also because of its fab colour. Beetroot is a good source of iron – which helps to carry oxygen around the blood – and vitamin C. It also contains nitrate, which gets converted into nitric oxide in the body. This also helps transport oxygen to every cell.

Serves 1

1 tablespoon olive oil
2 raw beetroots, diced
1 red onion, sliced
1 garlic clove, roughly chopped
2 new potatoes, diced
2 eggs
½ teaspoon paprika
salt and black pepper

1. Preheat the oven to 200°C (400°F), Gas Mark 6. Heat the oil in a small roasting tin in the oven, then add the beetroot and toss in the oil. Cook for 5 minutes, then add the onion, garlic and potatoes and mix to combine. Season to taste and cook for about 15 minutes, or until golden and tender, then remove from the oven.

2. Create two little wells in the veggies and crack an egg into each. Season well, sprinkle over the paprika and return to the oven. Cook for 10–15 minutes, or until the egg whites are set but the yolks are still runny. Serve immediately.

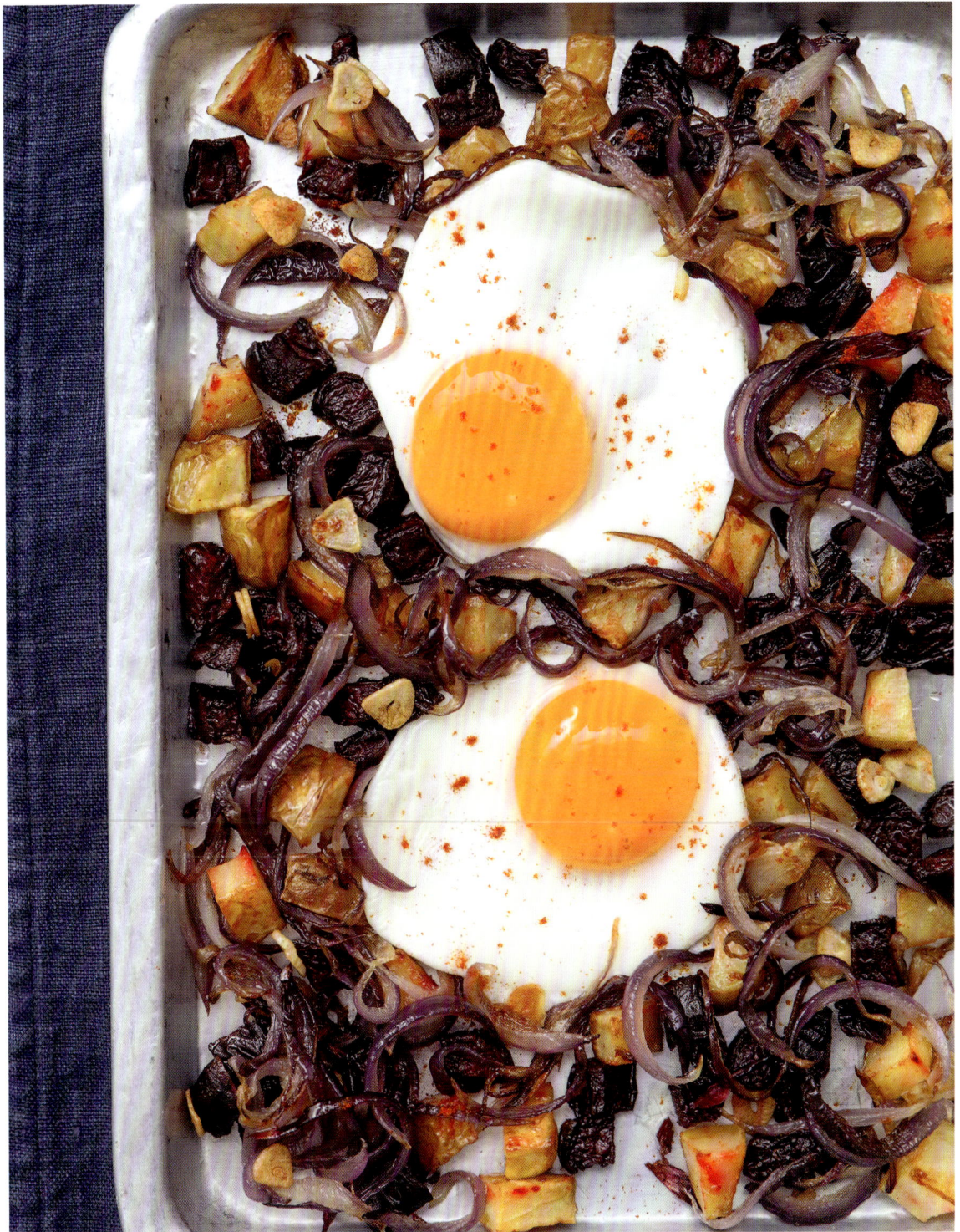

Raspberry & Chia Seed Pudding

Chia seeds are an excellent source of protein, fibre and omega-3 fatty acids, making this dish a super healthy start to the day.

Serves 1

50g (1¾oz) chia seeds
250ml (9fl oz) coconut milk
100g (3½oz) raspberries, plus extra
   to serve
2 tablespoons honey
1 tablespoon lemon juice
1 peach, pitted and sliced

1. Place the chia seeds and coconut milk in a bowl and stir well. Leave to soak for 5 minutes, stirring occasionally, until the seeds swell and thicken.

2. Place the raspberries, honey and lemon juice in a food processor and blitz until smooth.

3. Swirl the raspberry purée into the chia bowl and top with peach slices and a few extra raspberries.

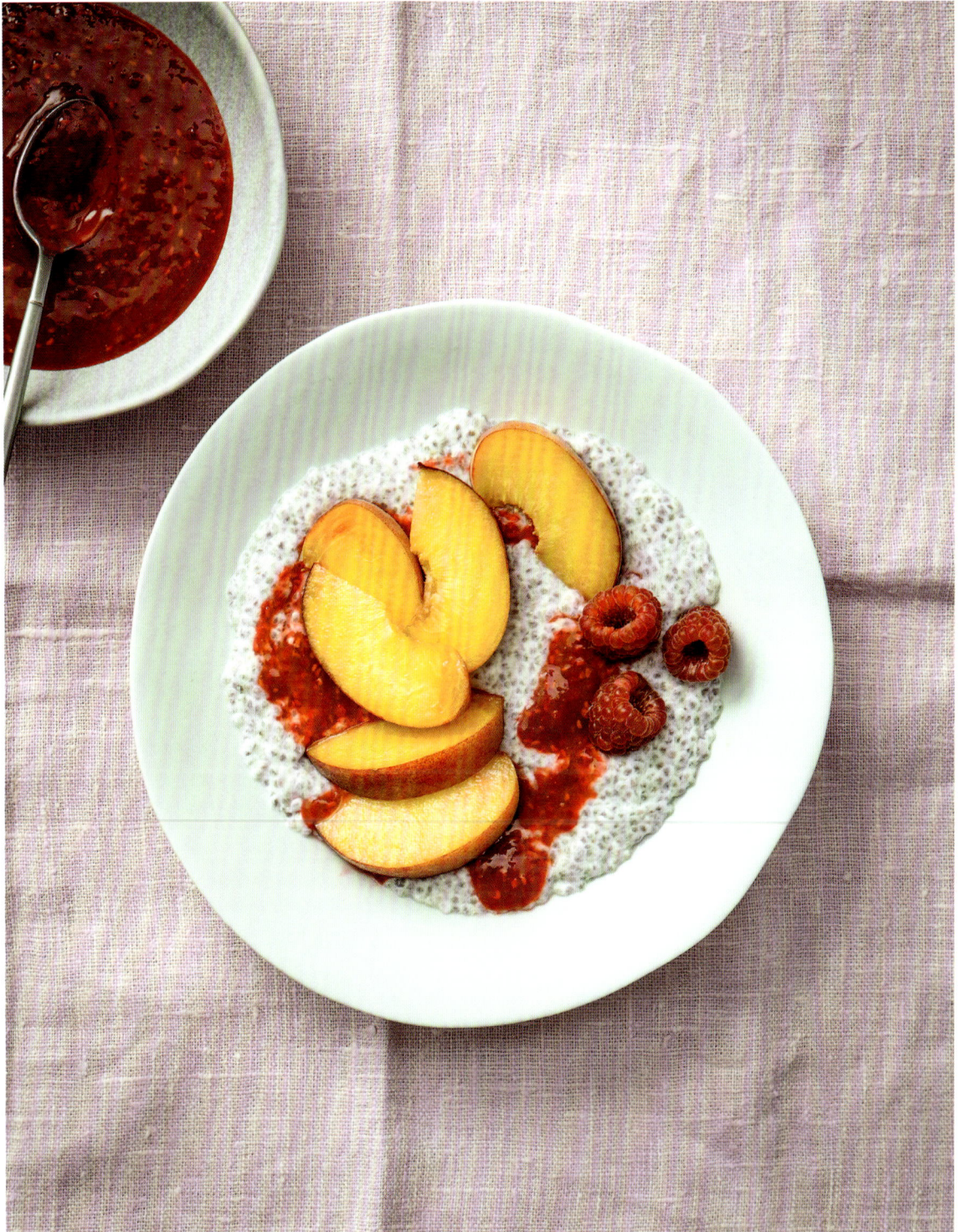

No-bake Chocolate Bars

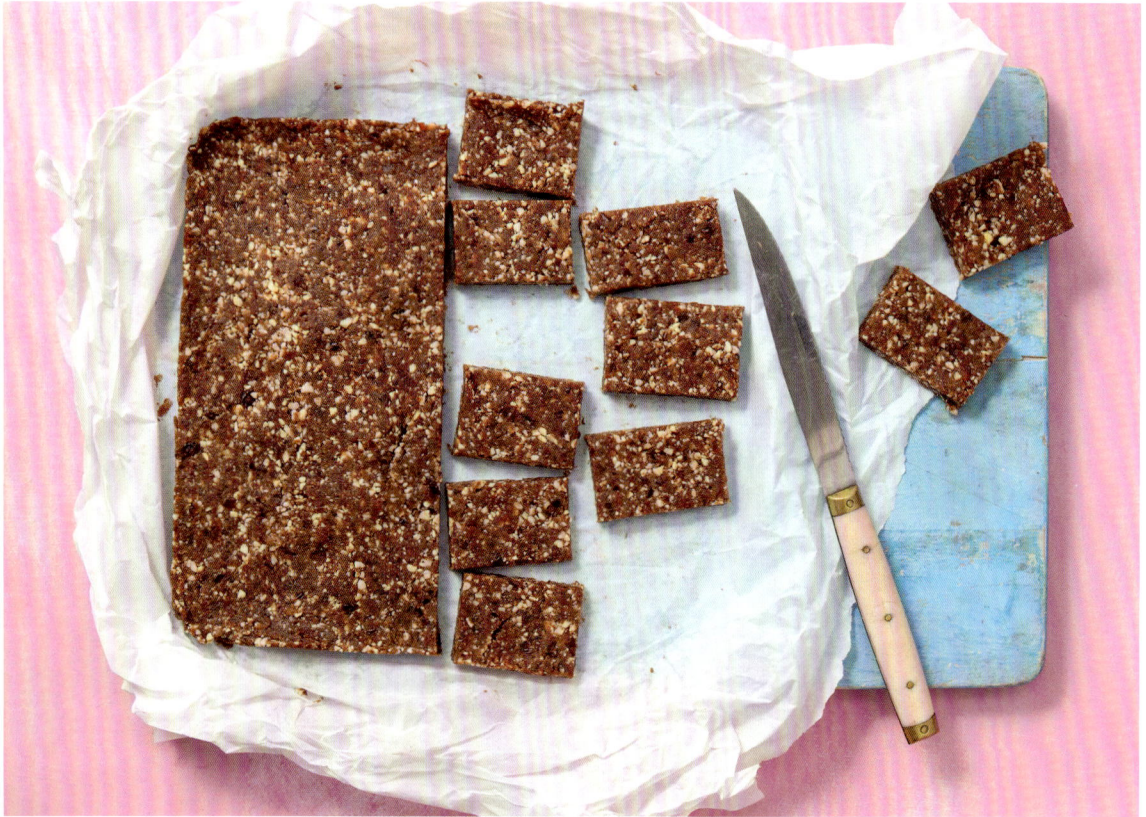

Makes 24

225g (8oz) medjool dates, pitted
150g (5½oz) cashew nuts
60g (2¼oz) ground almonds
1 heaped tablespoon cocoa powder
pinch of salt
1 tablespoon coconut oil

These delicious bars are super easy to make and a great snack for when you're on the go. I've made them with almonds and cashew nuts, both of which are good sources of vitamin E, which helps to protect our cells from oxidative damage. They also both contain high amounts of magnesium, which helps to relax our muscles and keep our blood sugars balanced.

1. Place all the ingredients, except the coconut oil, in a food processor and blitz until finely chopped and mixed together. Add the coconut oil and process for another minute until the mixture forms a squidgy dough.

2. Line a 20cm (8in) square baking tin with baking paper. Spoon the mixture into the tin and squish it into an even layer with your hands. Pop in the freezer for 30 minutes to firm up.

3. Cut into 24 bars. Store in an airtight container in the refrigerator for up to two weeks (they will also keep in the freezer for up to a month).

Chocolate Protein Balls

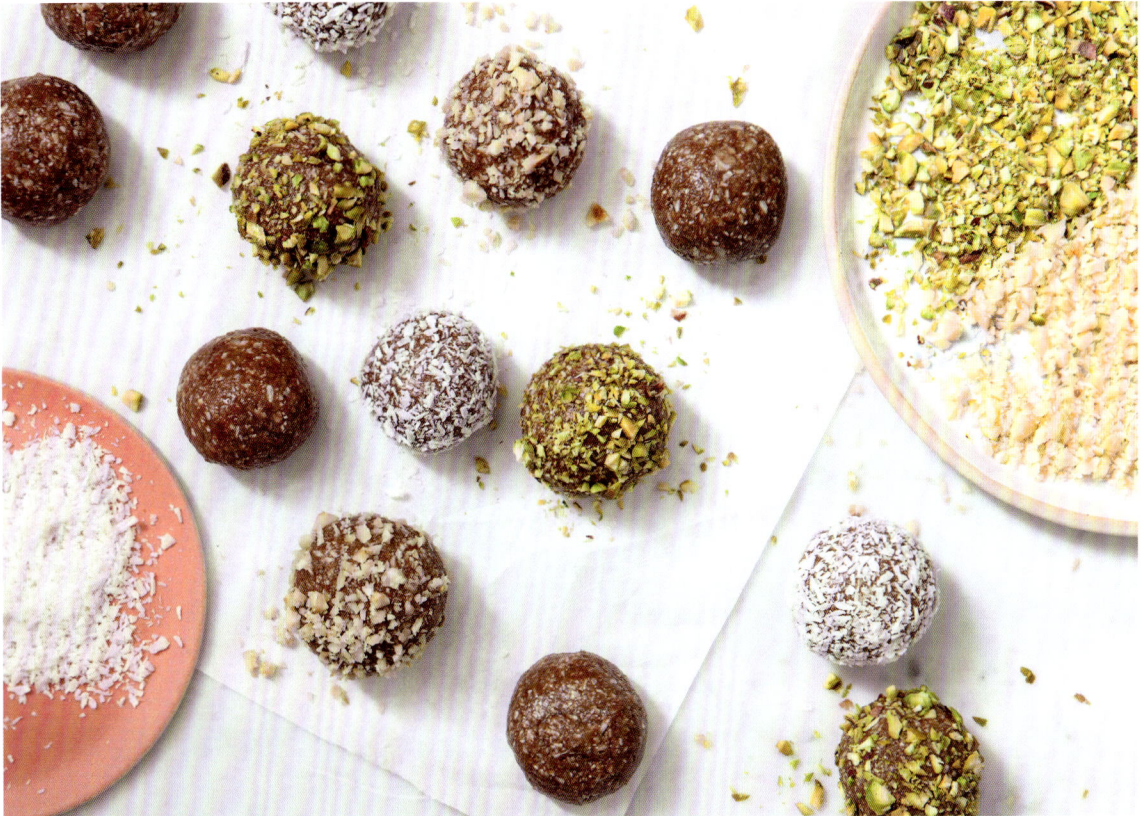

Makes 24

125g (4½oz) ground almonds
125g (4½oz) desiccated coconut
1 scoop or 20g (½oz) chocolate
   protein powder (see page 104)
1 tablespoon cocoa powder
125g (4½oz) honey
2 tablespoons coconut oil

For coating:
desiccated coconut
chopped pistachios
chopped almonds

I love these protein balls. They are quick to make and so versatile. Try swapping the cocoa powder for matcha or beetroot powder for a variety of flavours. Two of these protein balls make an excellent snack.

1. Place the ground almonds, coconut, protein powder and cocoa powder in a food processor and blitz until combined. Add the honey and coconut oil and process until the mixture forms a squidgy dough.

2. Using damp hands, roll the mixture into walnut-sized balls and pop in the refrigerator for at least 30 minutes to firm up. Roll some in desiccated coconut, some in chopped pistachios and some in chopped almonds and store in an airtight container for up to two weeks.

Coconut & Cranberry Energy Bars

One cup of cranberries gives you roughly 5g (⅛oz) of fibre.
They are also high in vitamin C and B vitamins which are required
for energy, so these bars are an excellent snack for a busy day.

<u>Makes 9</u>

90g (3¼oz) desiccated coconut
125g (4½oz) ground almonds
85g (3oz) oats
2 tablespoons honey
1 tablespoon coconut oil
125g (4½oz) dried cranberries

1. Place the coconut, almonds and oats in a food processor and blitz until finely chopped and mixed together. Add the honey and coconut oil and process for another minute until the mixture forms a squidgy dough. Stir in the cranberries.

2. Line a 20cm (8in) square baking tin with baking paper. Spoon the mixture into the tin and squish it into an even layer with your hands. Pop in the freezer for 30 minutes to firm up.

3. Cut into 9 bars. Store in an airtight container for up to two weeks.

<u>EVERYDAY HABITS THAT DRAIN OUR ENERGY:</u>

Taking things personally
Holding onto the past
Always checking Facebook
Over stressing
Skimping on sleep
Having a poor diet
Complaining all the time
Overthinking
Trying to please others
Not living in the moment

Let go of these habits, and you'll find you have more energy for the important things in your life.

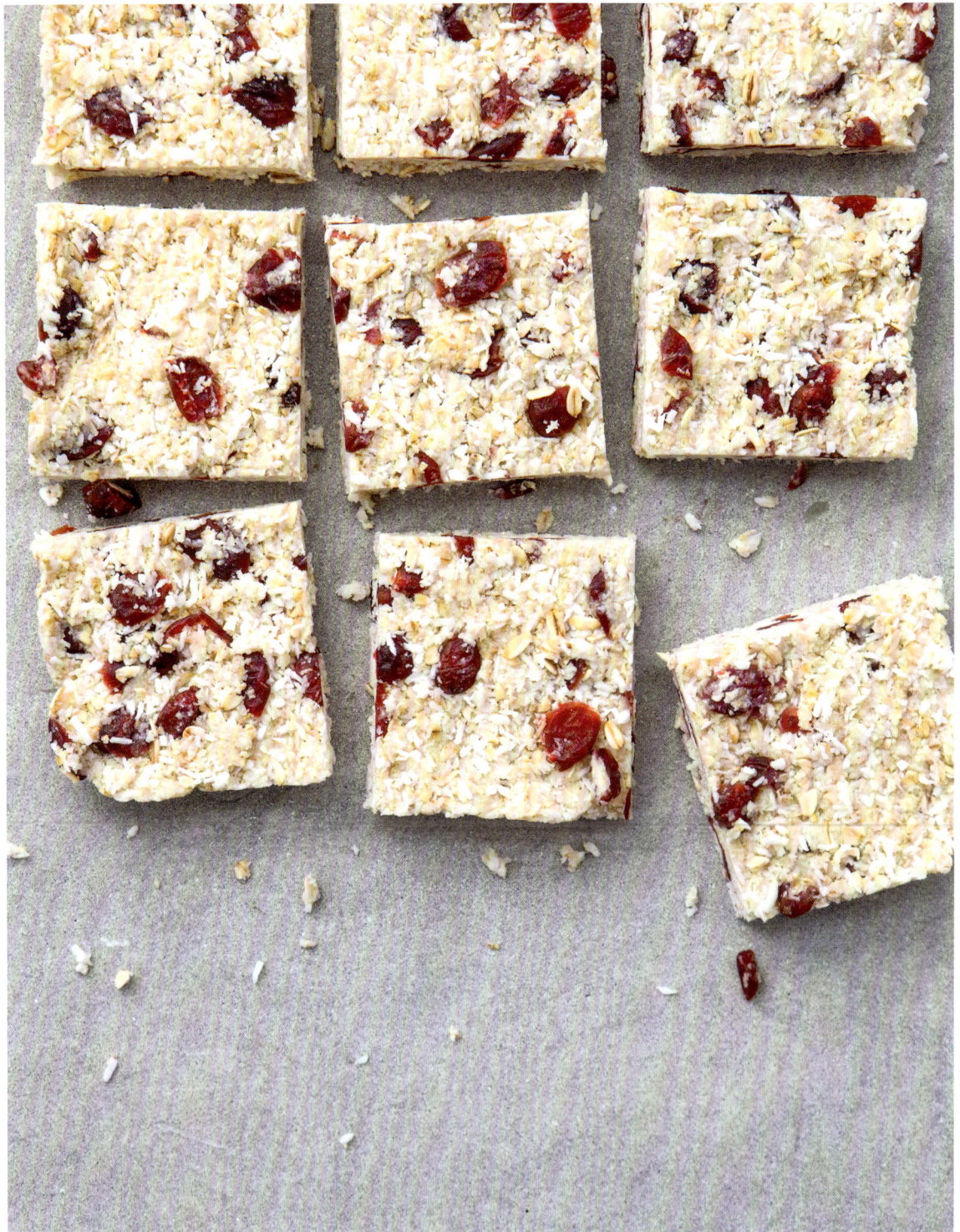

Matcha Balls

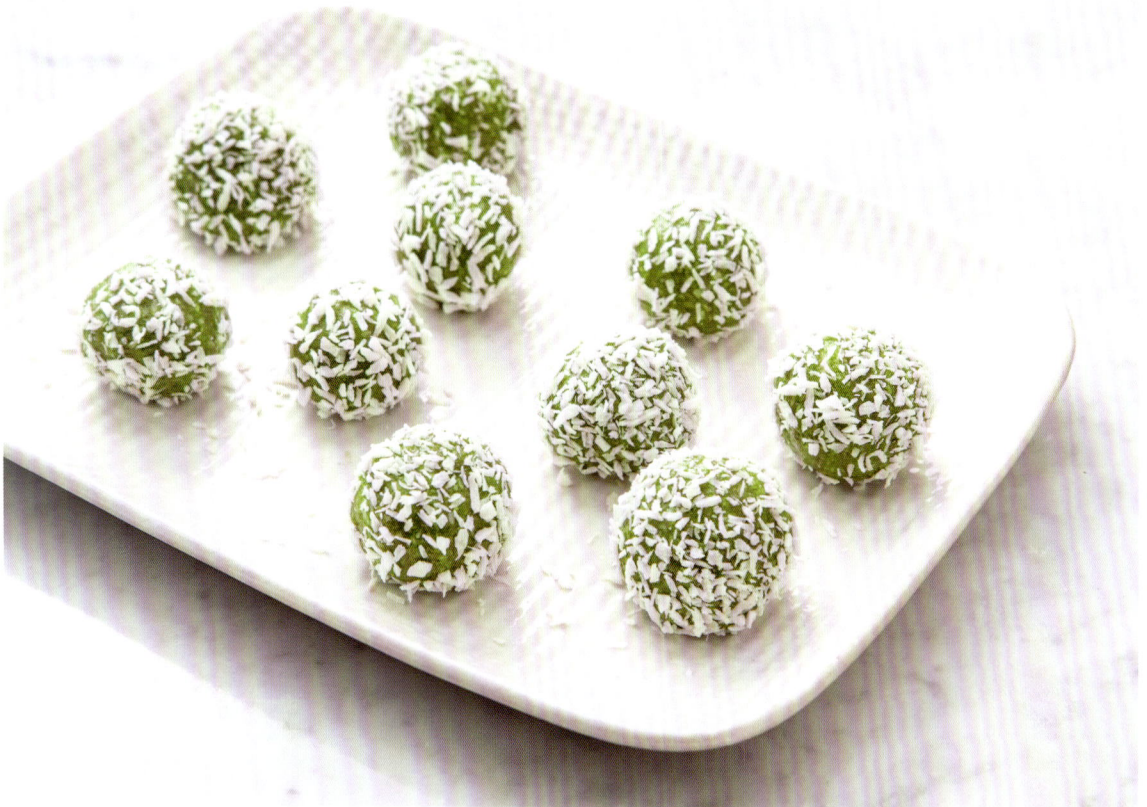

175g (6oz) desiccated coconut,
   plus extra for coating
1 scoop or 20g (½oz) vanilla protein
   powder (see page 104)
1 heaped tablespoon matcha powder
240g (8½oz) ground almonds
175–250g (6–9oz) honey
1 tablespoon coconut oil

These are my favourite snack because they look so vibrant and taste delicious. I've used matcha powder here but you can also use chocolate powder or beetroot powder to mix up the flavours.

1. Place the coconut, protein powder, matcha powder and almonds in a food processor and blitz until fully combined and powdery. Add 175g (6oz) of honey and the coconut oil and process for another 2–3 minutes. Check that the mixture clumps in your hand when you squeeze it – if not, add a little more honey.

2. Using damp hands, roll the mixture into walnut-sized balls and pop in the refrigerator for at least 30 minutes to firm up. Roll in desiccated coconut, and store in an airtight container for up to two weeks.

Chickpea Protein Bars

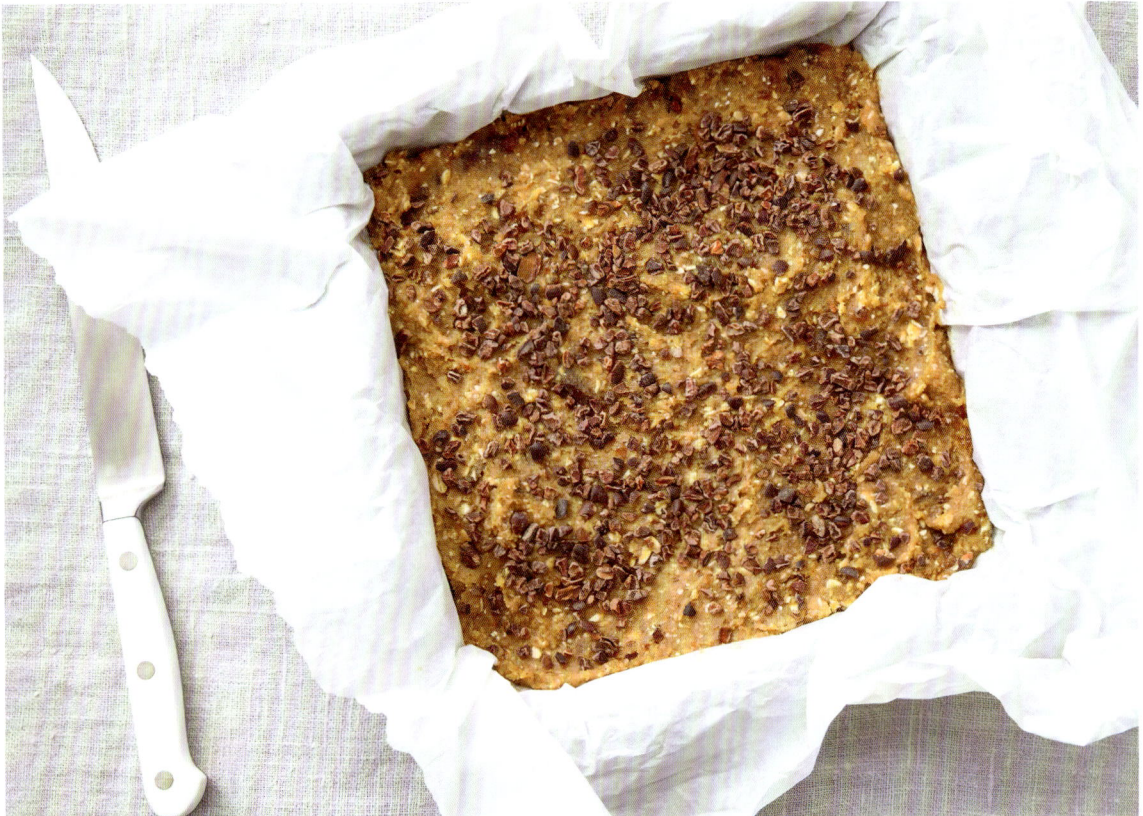

Makes 12

400g (14oz) can chickpeas, rinsed
    and drained
85g (3oz) oats
60g (2¼oz) ground almonds
2 scoops or 40g (1oz) vanilla protein
    powder (see page 104)
2 tablespoons peanut butter
16 medjool dates, pitted
1 tablespoon almond milk
cacao nibs, for sprinkling

I loooveee these bars. The chickpeas provide the protein, as does the additional protein powder. The dates and oats provide the fibre and B vitamins. And the results taste like healthy fudge!

1. Place all the ingredients, except the cacao nibs, in a food processor and blitz until you have a dough-like mixture.

2. Line a 20cm (8in) square baking tin with baking paper. Spoon the mixture into the tin and spread it into an even layer. Sprinkle the cacao nibs on top and press them in with your fingers. Pop in the refrigerator for 1 hour to firm up.

3. Cut into 12 bars. Store in an airtight container in the refrigerator for up to a week.

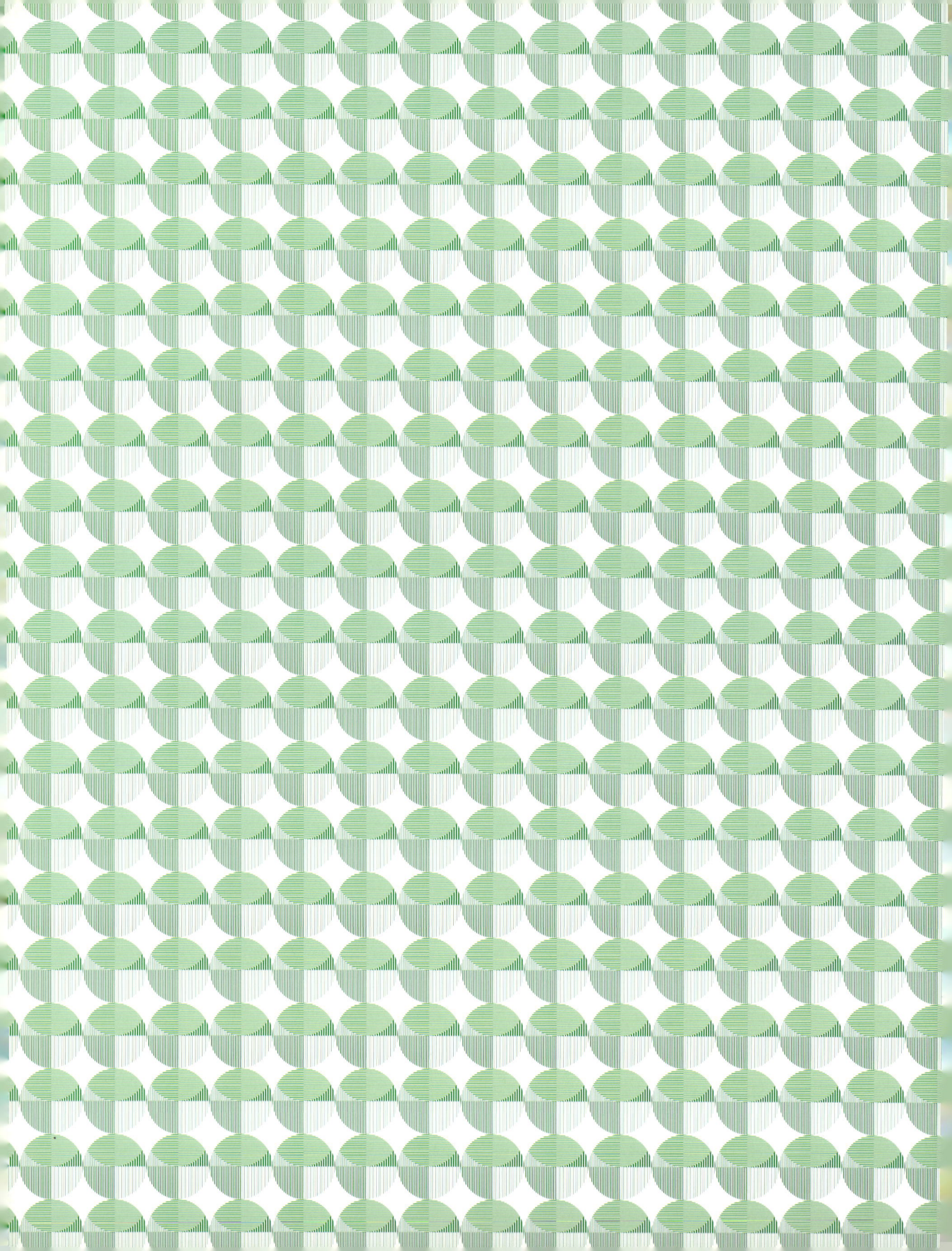

Lunch

Glow Bowl

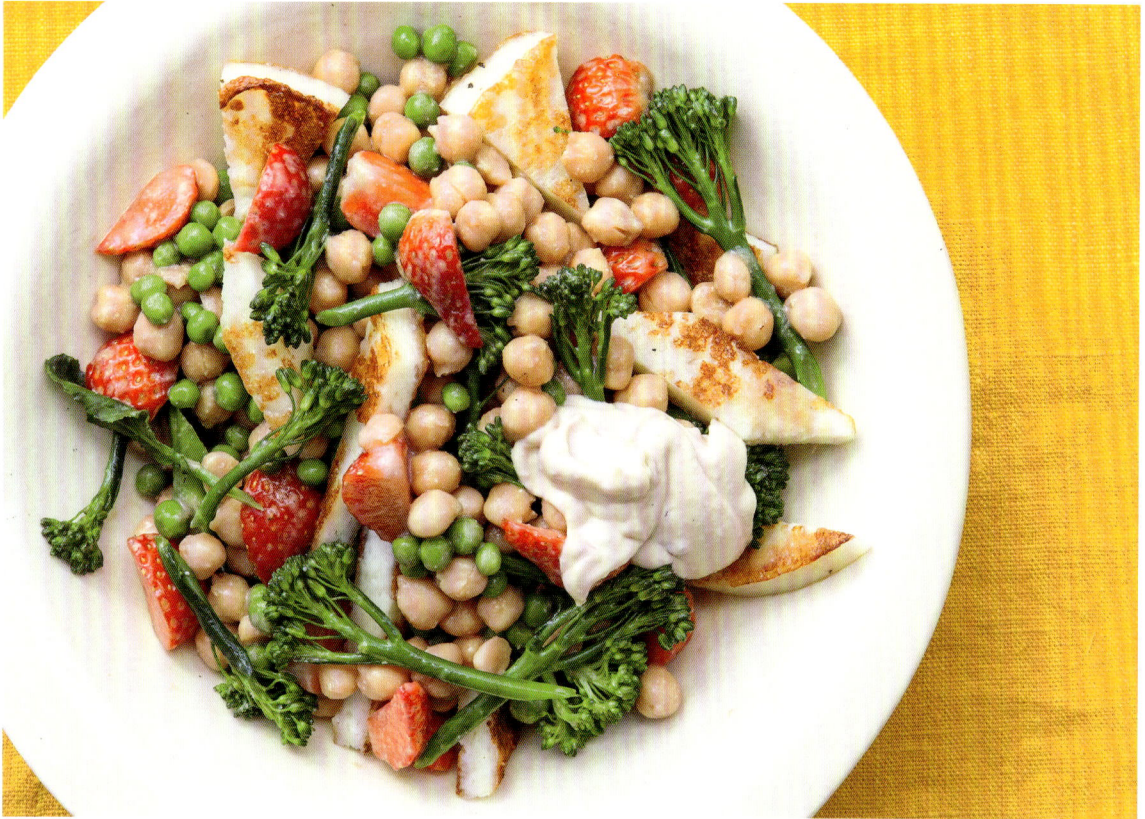

Serves 1

200g (7oz) canned chickpeas,
    drained and rinsed
handful of broccoli spears, cooked
    and cooled
handful of peas, cooked and cooled
10 strawberries, chopped
1 teaspoon olive oil
4 slices of halloumi
dollop of hummus, to serve

For the Miso dressing:
1 tablespoon miso paste
1 tablespoon soy sauce
1 tablespoon rice vinegar
1 tablespoon sesame oil

This glow bowl is a great way to pack a lot of nutrients into a dish quickly! I've used strawberries since they are one of my magnificent seven and I've also added halloumi, which is a great source of protein.

1. Place the dressing ingredients in a serving bowl and whisk to combine. Add the chickpeas, broccoli, peas and strawberries and toss lightly to coat.

2. Heat the oil in a frying pan over a high heat, add the halloumi and cook for 1–2 minutes on each side until golden. Chop and stir into the salad. Top with a dollop of hummus.

Sesame Soba Noodle Salad

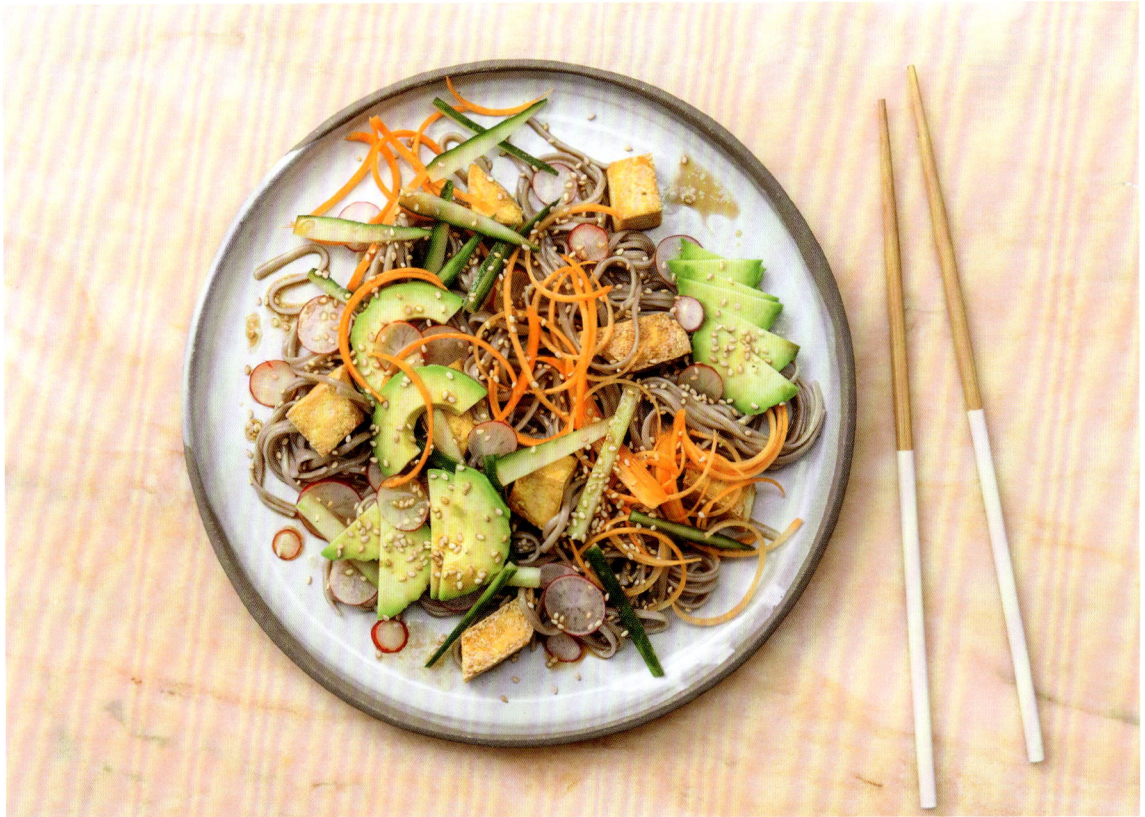

Serves 1

1 bundle of soba noodles
250g (9oz) precooked or raw firm
   tofu, diced
2 radishes, finely sliced
½ carrot, peeled and cut into
   matchsticks
½ cucumber, cut into matchsticks
½ avocado, chopped
1 tablespoon sesame seeds (black,
   white or a mixture)

For the dressing:
2 teaspoons sesame oil
2 teaspoons soy sauce
1 teaspoon rice wine vinegar
1 teaspoon lime juice
½ teaspoon honey

Soba noodles are usually made from buckwheat, making them gluten free. They a good source of fibre, B1 and manganese and are super quick and easy to cook.

1. Cook the soba noodles according to packet instructions. Drain and rinse thoroughly in cold water as soba noodles have a tendency to stick together.

2. If your tofu needs cooking, heat 1 teaspoon of the sesame oil in a nonstick frying pan over a medium-high heat and cook the tofu, stirring regularly, until golden all over.

3. Meanwhile, place all the dressing ingredients in a large bowl and whisk to combine. Add the radishes, carrot and cucumber and toss to coat in the dressing, then add the tofu and noodles and toss again.

4. Transfer to a plate and top with the avocado and the sesame seeds.

Greek Pasta Salad with Quick Pickled Red Onions

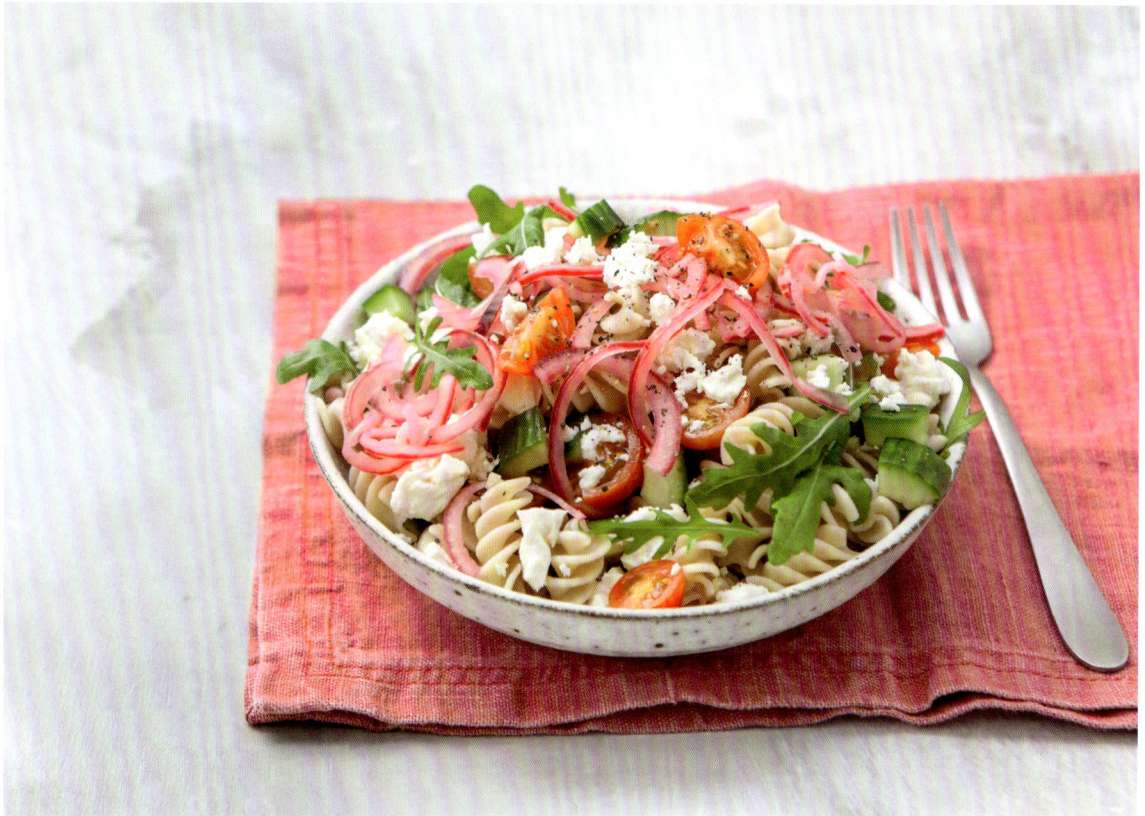

<u>Serves 1</u>

75g (2¾oz) brown rice pasta
1 small red onion, finely sliced
2 tablespoons red or white wine
   vinegar
handful of cherry tomatoes, halved
½ cucumber, diced
handful of rocket
olive oil, for drizzling
balsamic vinegar, for drizzling
50g (1¾oz) feta
salt and black pepper

Brown rice pasta is a great source of carbohydrates, so this is an energy-dense dish.

1. Cook the pasta in a saucepan of lightly salted boiling water according to packet instructions. While it's cooking, mix the onion and vinegar in a shallow bowl and set aside.

2. Place the tomatoes, cucumber and rocket in a serving bowl. Once the pasta is cooked, drain well and rinse in cold water. Add to the bowl with a good drizzle of olive oil, a drizzle of balsamic vinegar and a good pinch of seasoning.

3. Drain the onion – it should have turned bright pink – and add to the bowl. Toss everything together, then crumble the feta on top.

Chickpea, Avocado & Feta Salad

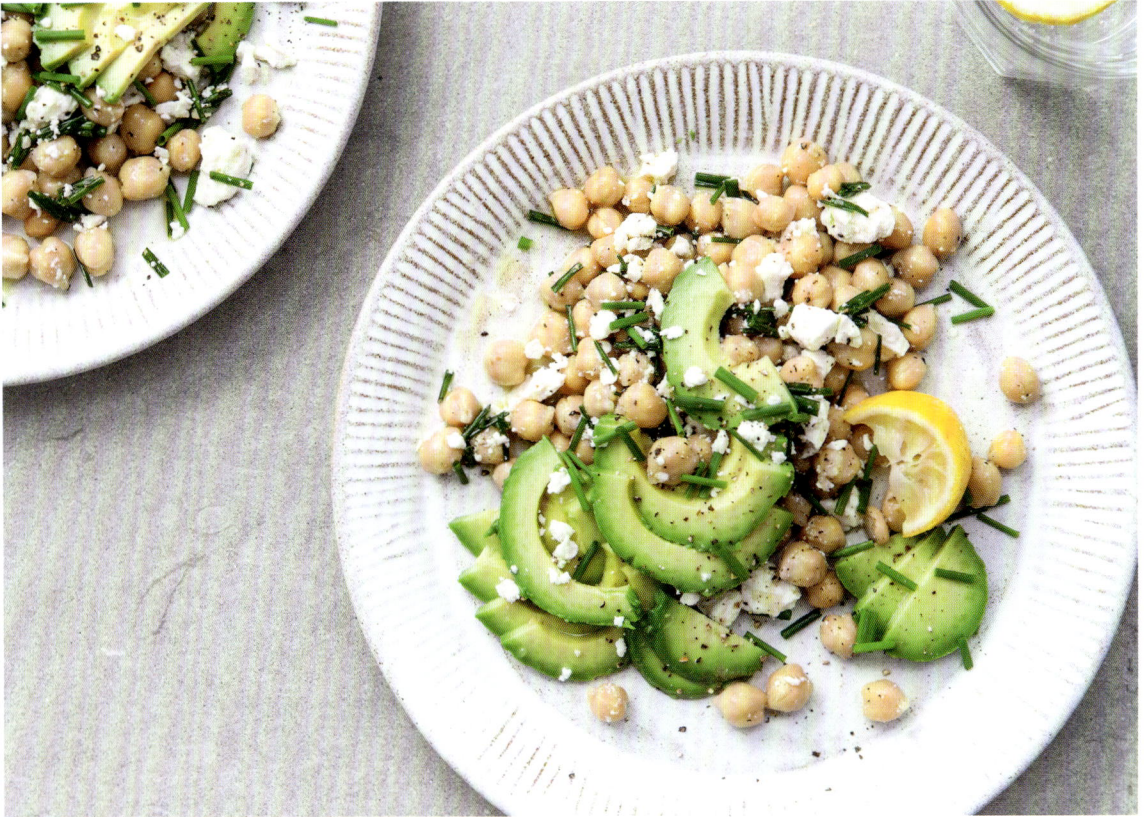

Serves 1

400g (14oz) can chickpeas, rinsed
  and drained
½ avocado, chopped
50g (1¾oz) feta cheese
handful of chopped chives
olive oil, for drizzling
salt and black pepper

Chickpeas are an excellent source of plant protein, and because of their fibre and nutrient profile, they also help to keep blood sugar levels balanced. Plus, they are extremely versatile and inexpensive!

1. Place the chickpeas, avocado, feta and chives in a large serving bowl. Season to taste, drizzle with olive oil and mix to combine.

Mexican Brown Rice Rainbow Bowl

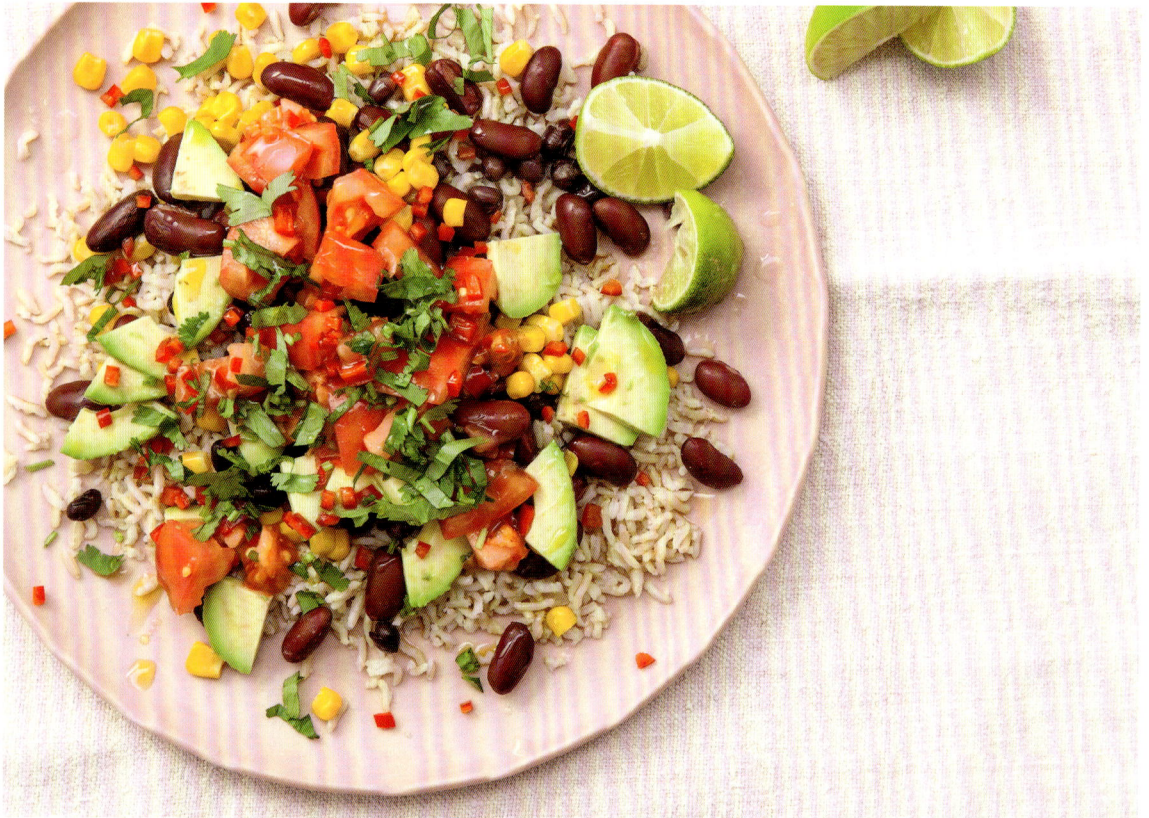

Serves 1

150g (5½oz) cooked brown rice
200g (7oz) canned sweetcorn
70g (2½oz) canned black beans,
   adzuki beans or kidney beans,
   drained and rinsed
½ avocado, diced
1 tablespoon lime juice
olive oil, for drizzling
salt and black pepper
crumbled feta, to serve (optional)

Tomato salsa
1 large tomato, diced
½ red chilli, finely chopped
1 tablespoon chopped coriander
1 tablespoon lime juice

Brown rice has a low glycaemic index. This means that it releases sugars into the blood stream slowly, providing you with sustainable energy. It's also a good source of fibre and magnesium.

1. Mix all the salsa ingredients together in a small bowl and season well.

2. Place the brown rice in a serving bowl and top with the sweetcorn, beans, avocado and then the tomato salsa. Mix the lime juice with a drizzle of olive oil, season and then dress your bowl. Top with crumbled feta, if using.

Prawn & Courgette Bowl with Watercress Dressing

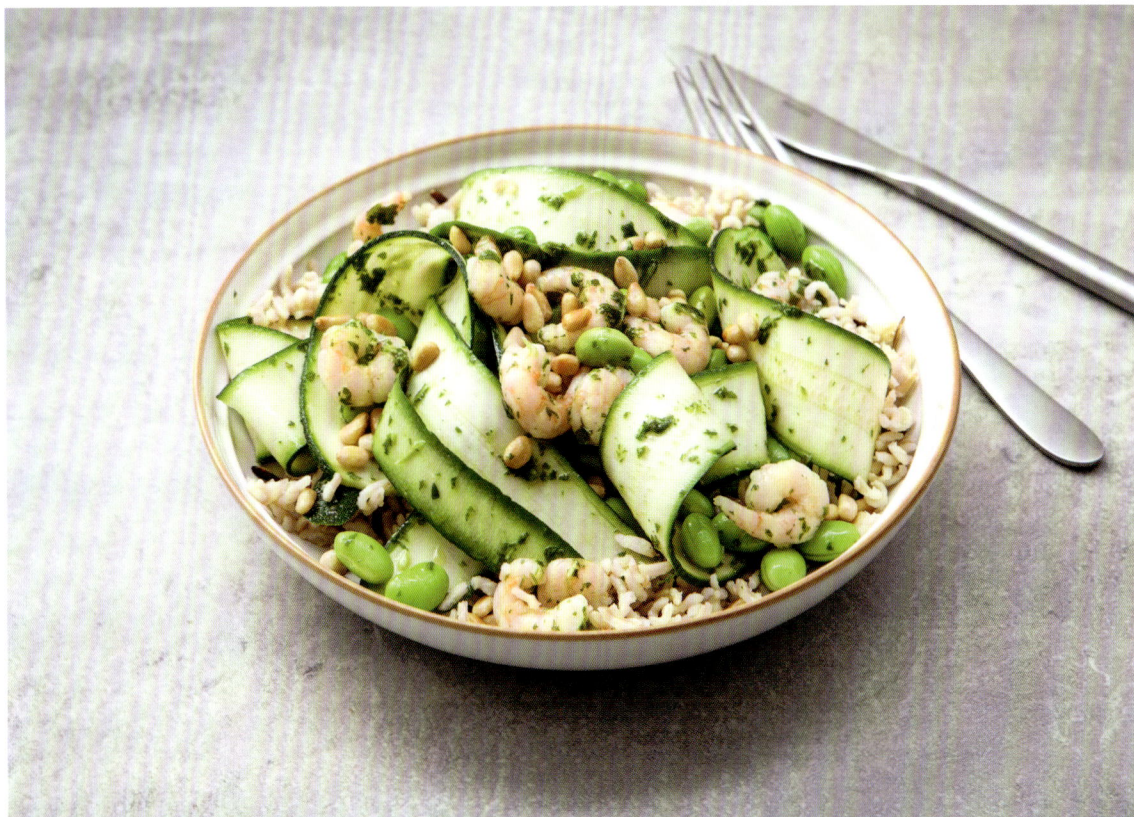

<u>Serves 1</u>

2 teaspoons pine nuts
1 courgette
150g (5½oz) cooked peeled prawns
handful of edamame beans
brown rice, wild rice or quinoa,
   to serve

For the dressing:
handful of watercress
2 tablespoons olive oil
1 tablespoon white wine vinegar
salt and black pepper

I love watercress! It's packed with magnesium and iron, and also has good levels of vitamin K.

1. Place the dressing ingredients in a food processor and blitz until smooth.

2. Place the pine nuts in a dry frying pan over a medium heat and toast, stirring constantly, until golden.

3. Use a vegetable peeler to shave the courgette into long, wide ribbons and place in a large bowl. Add the prawns, edamame beans, pine nuts and dressing, toss to coat and serve with the wholegrain of your choice.

Smoked Mackerel, Beetroot & Watercress Salad

This salad is delicious and so easy to make – perfect for when you are feeling super tired or are short on time. I've included watercress because it is a good source of magnesium and iron, both of which are needed for energy.

Serves 1

1 large smoked mackerel fillet,
  skinned and flaked
3 small cooked beetroots, quartered
½ avocado, sliced
125g (4½oz) cooked Puy lentils
large handful of watercress

For the dressing:
2 teaspoons creamed horseradish
1 teaspoon Dijon mustard
1 tablespoon olive oil
juice of ½ lemon
black pepper

1. Place the dressing ingredients in a serving bowl, season with pepper and whisk to combine. Add all the salad ingredients and toss lightly to coat.

REMEMBER...

Food in is energy in.

So please don't skip meals. If you're extremely tired and don't have much energy to cook, go for one of the simpler recipes, such as this salad or the Avocado & Feta Pitta Pockets on page 158. These recipes take just minutes to prepare.

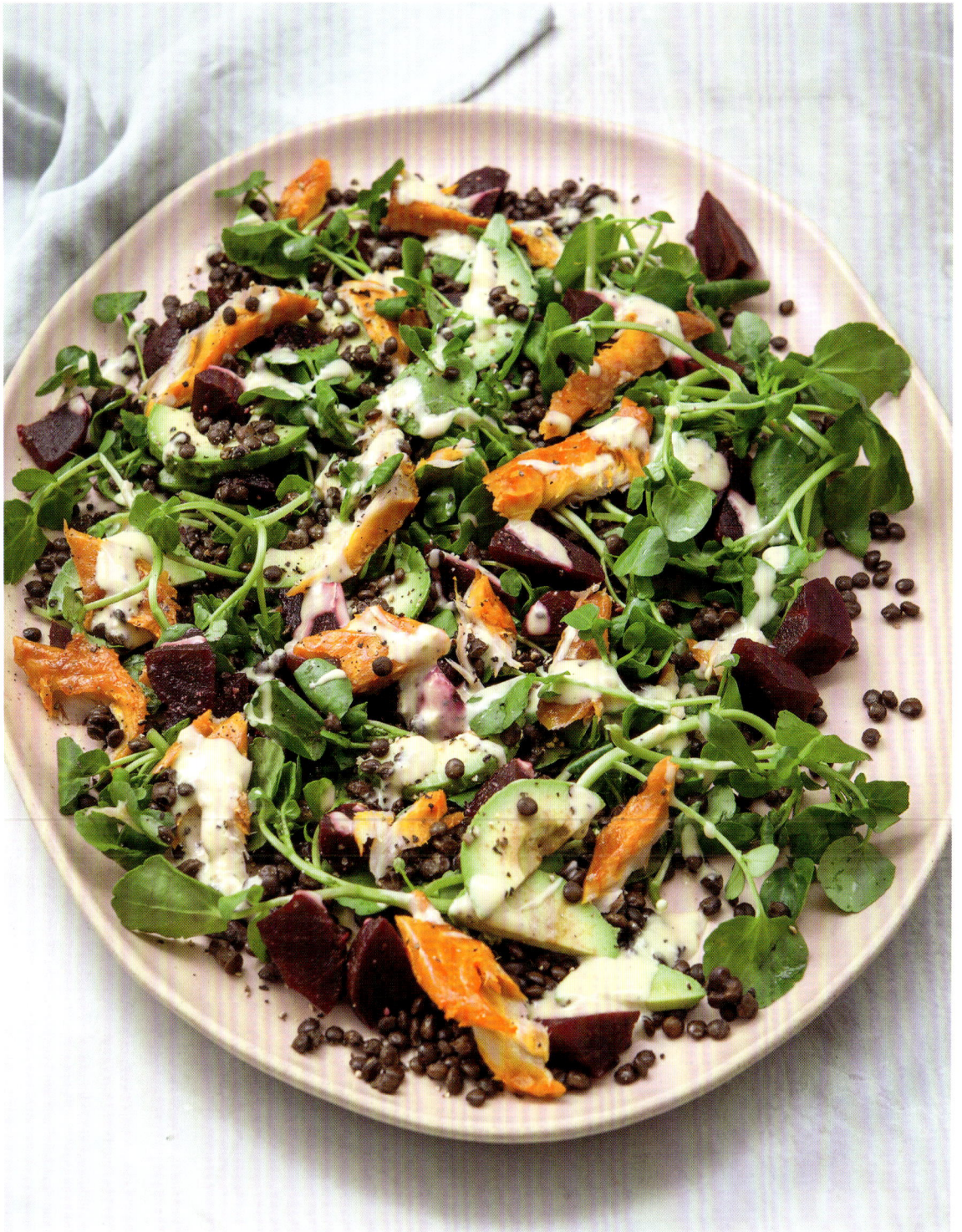

Prawn & Corn Salad

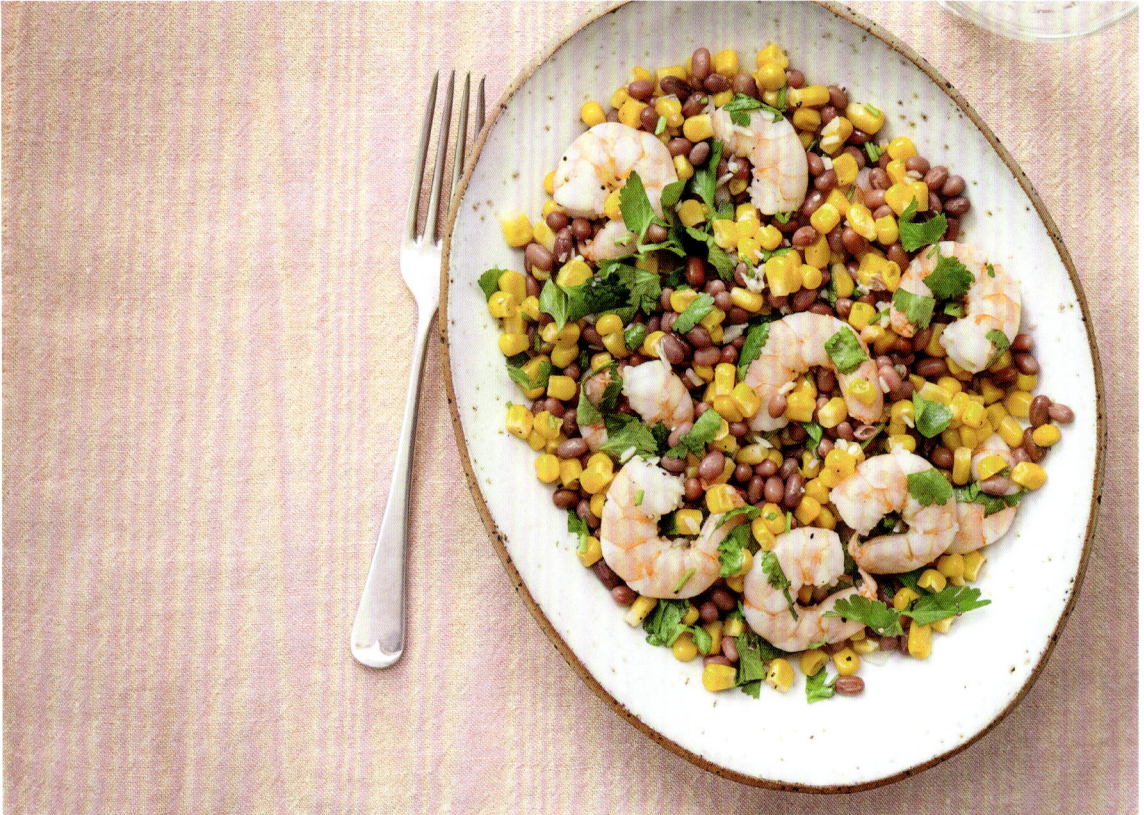

Serves 1

knob of butter
2 garlic cloves, crushed
juice of 1 lemon
100g (3½oz) cooked peeled king
    prawns
160g (5¾oz) canned sweetcorn
200g (7oz) canned adzuki or mung
    beans, rinsed and drained
handful of chopped coriander, plus
    extra to serve
salt and black pepper

I love this combo! It creates a nice, meaty dish that is filling and packed with nutrients. It's super quick to make, and the beans are an excellent source of B vitamins, which are essential for energy, so this dish is great for when you are feeling especially tired.

1. Melt the butter in a frying pan over a medium-high heat, add the garlic, lemon juice and prawns and cook, stirring, for about 5 minutes or until heated through.

2. Mix the corn and beans together in a bowl and add the coriander. Add the prawns and any cooking liquid, season to taste and toss together. Serve garnished with extra coriander.

Simple Salmon Salad

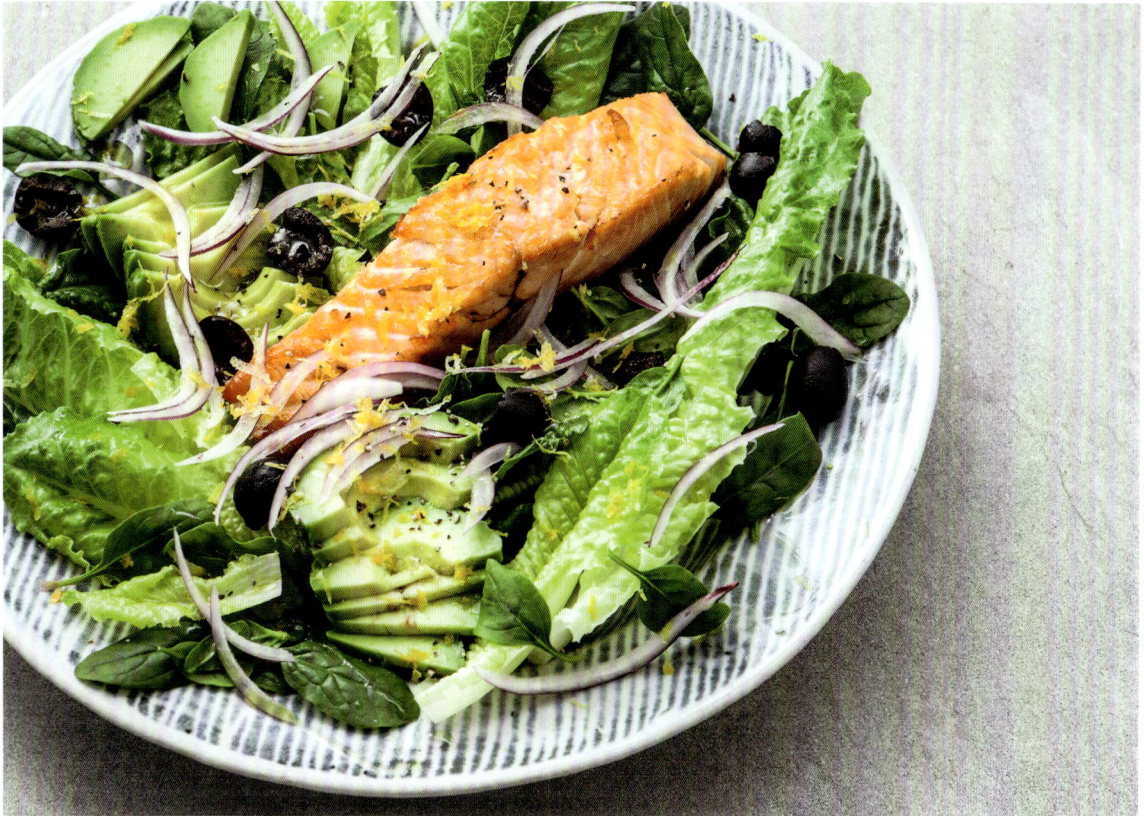

Serves 1

knob of butter (optional)
1 raw or cooked salmon fillet
½ Romaine lettuce, divided into leaves
handful of baby spinach
½ red onion, sliced
5–10 black olives, halved
½ avocado, sliced
lemon juice, to taste
olive oil, for drizzling
black pepper

Salmon is an excellent source of protein, omega-3 fatty acids, selenium, vitamin A and vitamin D. All perfect for supporting our immune system.

1. If using raw salmon, melt the butter in a frying pan over a medium heat, add the salmon and cook for 3–5 minutes on each side until cooked to your liking.

2. Arrange the lettuce and spinach on a plate and top with the onion, olives, avocado and salmon. Drizzle with lemon juice and olive oil and season with black pepper.

Salmon & Pear Salad

*I love adding fruit to salads to give them another level of flavour.
The sweet hit from the pear makes this dish more exciting,
while also packing in more nutrients.*

Serves 1

handful of pine nuts or walnuts
knob of butter
1 salmon fillet
lemon juice, to taste
large handful of rocket
1 pear, cored and sliced
2 tablespoons shop-bought honey
   and mustard dressing
Salt and black pepper
pomegranate seeds, to decorate

1. Place the pine nuts or walnuts in a dry frying pan over a medium heat and toast, stirring constantly, until golden. Remove from the pan and set aside.

2. Melt the butter in the frying pan over a medium heat, add the salmon and cook for 3–5 minutes on each side until cooked to your liking. Squeeze over some lemon juice, season to taste and set aside.

3. Assemble the salad by arranging the rocket on a plate, followed by the sliced pear. Flake the salmon over the salad, then sprinkle the nuts on top. Drizzle with the dressing and finish with a handful of pomegranate seeds for a pop of colour and extra vitamin C.

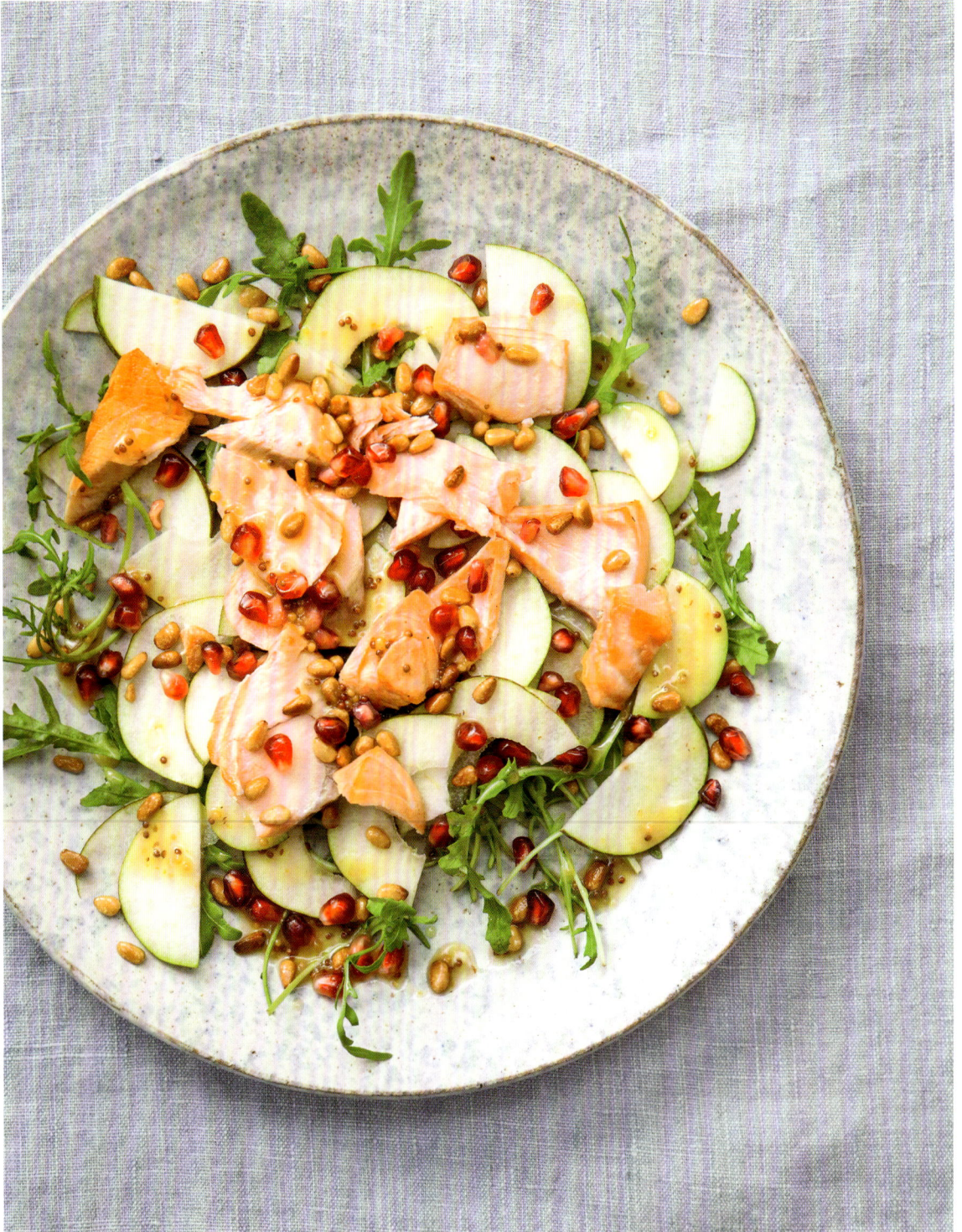

Raw Vegan Sushi

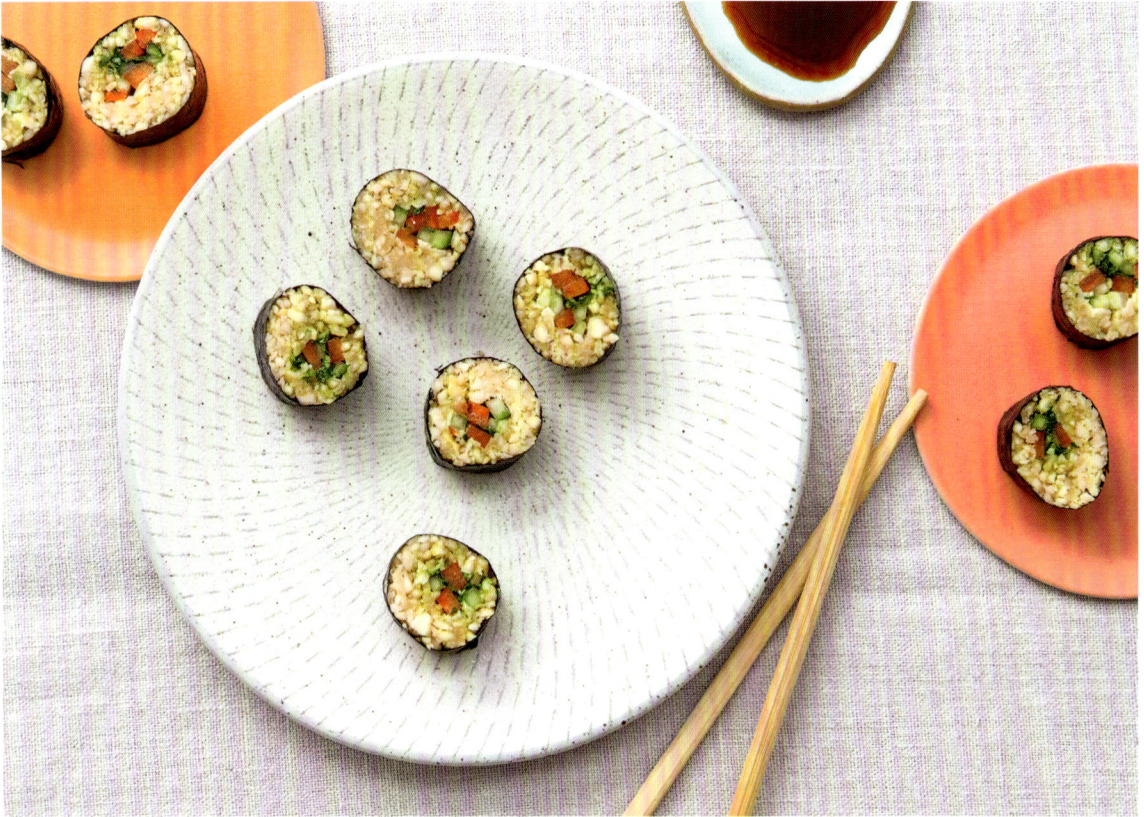

<u>Serves 2</u>

300g (10½oz) cashew nuts
2 garlic cloves, crushed
1 tablespoon rice vinegar
3 tablespoons olive oil
2 sheets of nori seaweed
1 red pepper, cored, deseeded
   and cut into matchsticks
½ cucumber, cut into matchsticks
soy sauce, for dipping

I've used cashew nuts here instead of rice, to make this dish more nutrient dense and filling. The nori is an excellent source of iodine and selenium, both of which support the thyroid gland.

1. Place the cashews in a food processor and blitz until the pieces are the size of rice grains. Add the garlic, vinegar and oil and pulse until well combined.

2. Lay out the sheets of nori and divide the nut mixture between them, arranging it in an even layer to cover two-thirds of each sheet. Lay the sticks of pepper and cucumber in a line down the middle of the nut mixture.

3. Lightly wet the uncovered portion of the seaweed with a little water and roll up the sushi rolls. Start rolling at the nut end, enclosing the pepper and cucumber pieces, and finish with the dampened seaweed to wrap around the roll and stick it together. Cut each of the rolls into 6 or 8 pieces and serve with soy sauce for dipping.

Seared Tuna Wraps with Matcha Dip

<u>Serves 2</u>

1 teaspoon olive oil
1 fresh tuna steak
rice paper wraps
½ carrot, peeled and cut into matchsticks
½ cucumber, cut into matchsticks
1 spring onion, finely sliced

Matcha dip
½ avocado
1 teaspoon matcha powder
1 teaspoon honey or maple syrup
1 tablespoon olive oil
1 tablespoon rice wine vinegar
1–2 tablespoons water
salt and black pepper

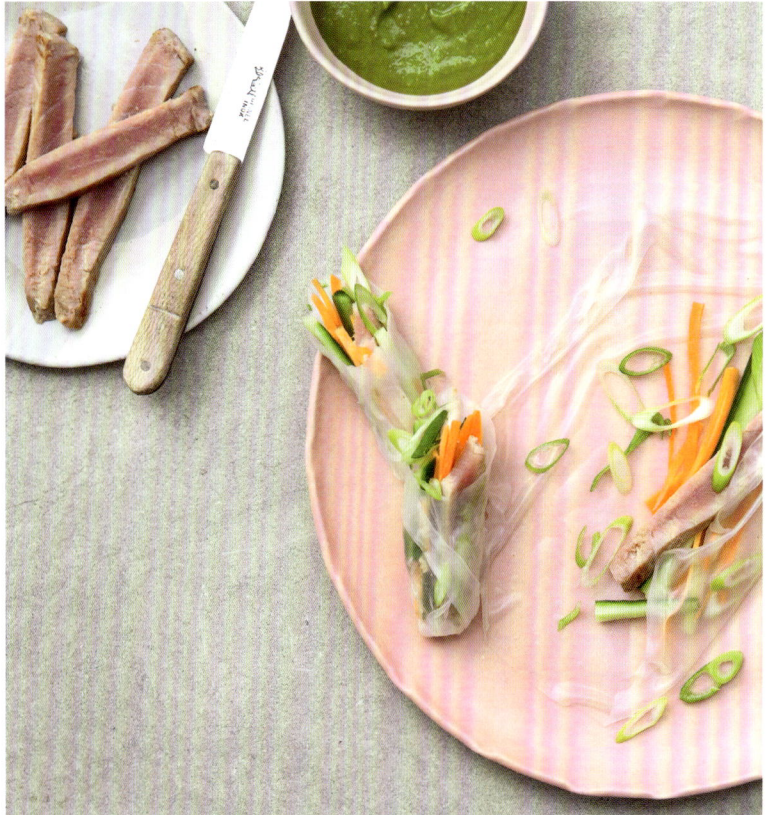

Tuna contains good amounts of zinc and selenium, both of which support the thyroid gland and the immune system.

1. Heat the oil in a nonstick frying pan over a medium-high heat, season the tuna steak well on both sides, then cook for 1–2 minutes until golden underneath. Tuna cooks really quickly, so keep your eye on it. Turn it over, and when the top and bottom are cooked but you can still see a pink line running through the middle, it's ready. Slice it thinly and set to one side.

2. Place all the dip ingredients in a food processor, season to taste and blitz until smooth, adding a little more water or vinegar if it's very thick. Transfer to a small bowl.

3. Prepare the rice paper wraps according to packet instructions. Most need to be soaked in cold water for 1–2 minutes. Lay out the soaked wraps and start layering up the tuna slices and veggies on top. Fold any way you like to seal – triangular parcels or rolls both work well – and dip away.

Beetroot Falafel with Green Quinoa Salad

Who doesn't love falafel? I've added beetroot to give this dish a vibrant colour, and because they are one of my magnificent seven ingredients (see page 49).

Serves 4

400g (14oz) can chickpeas, rinsed
   and drained
2 raw beetroots, diced
1 teaspoon paprika
1 teaspoon ground cumin
1 tablespoon gluten-free flour
1 teaspoon sesame seeds (black,
   white or a mixture)
salt and black pepper

For the salad
250g (9oz) pack of ready-cooked
   quinoa
handful of chopped mint leaves
handful of chopped coriander leaves
1 spring onion, finely sliced
handful of edamame beans
½ cucumber, diced

For the dressing:
1 tablespoon good-quality tahini
juice of 1 lemon
1 teaspoon maple syrup

1. Preheat the oven to 190°C (375°F), Gas Mark 5, and line a baking tray with baking paper.

Place the chickpeas, beetroots, paprika and cumin in a food processor and blitz until the mixture forms a paste. Season to taste, add the flour and blend again until the mixture is firm enough to roll into balls. If necessary, add a little more flour to stiffen, or a little water to loosen the mixture.

2. Using damp hands, form the mixture into 12 balls about the size of golf balls and place them on the lined baking tray. Sprinkle with the sesame seeds, then cook for about 25 minutes, or until crisp.

3. For the salad, combine all the ingredients in a bowl, season well and transfer to a serving plate.

4. For the dressing, whisk together the ingredients in a small bowl with a pinch of salt, adding a little warm water to loosen it. Don't worry if it starts off a bit grainy, just keep on whisking and adding a little more water if necessary; it can take a few minutes to get to the right consistency. It should ending up looking like mayonnaise.

5. Serve the falafels on top of the salad, with the tahini dressing.

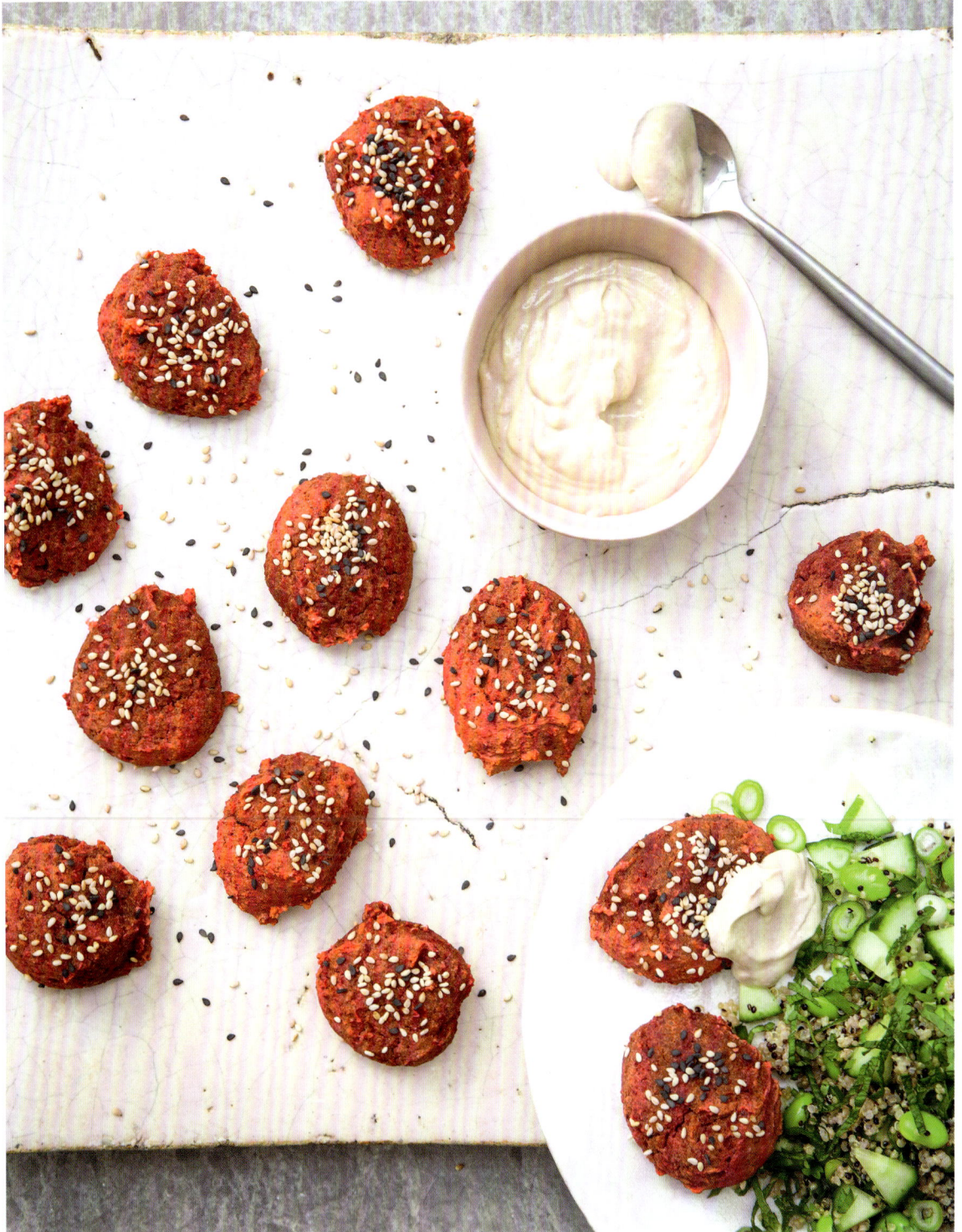

Mango, Chicken & Cashew Salad

I've added mango to this chicken salad to give it a bit of a tangy kick. Mango is an excellent source of vitamins A and C, as well as a good source of fibre.

Serves 1

handful of cashew nuts
½ mango, not too ripe, chopped
½ avocado, sliced
2 spring onions, chopped
handful of coriander leaves
handful of baby spinach
1 cooked chicken breast, sliced
olive oil, for drizzling
juice of ½ lime
salt and black pepper

1. Place the cashews in a dry frying pan over a medium heat and toast, stirring constantly, until golden.

2. Place all the ingredients in a serving bowl, drizzle with olive oil and lime juice, season to taste and toss together.

TOP TIP

'If you're tired, learn to rest. Not quit.'

If you're feeling really exhausted today and just need to sleep, then sleep.

Listen to your body and nap when it needs to. Ask someone to come over and cook or order something healthy for when you wake up. Rest is productive.

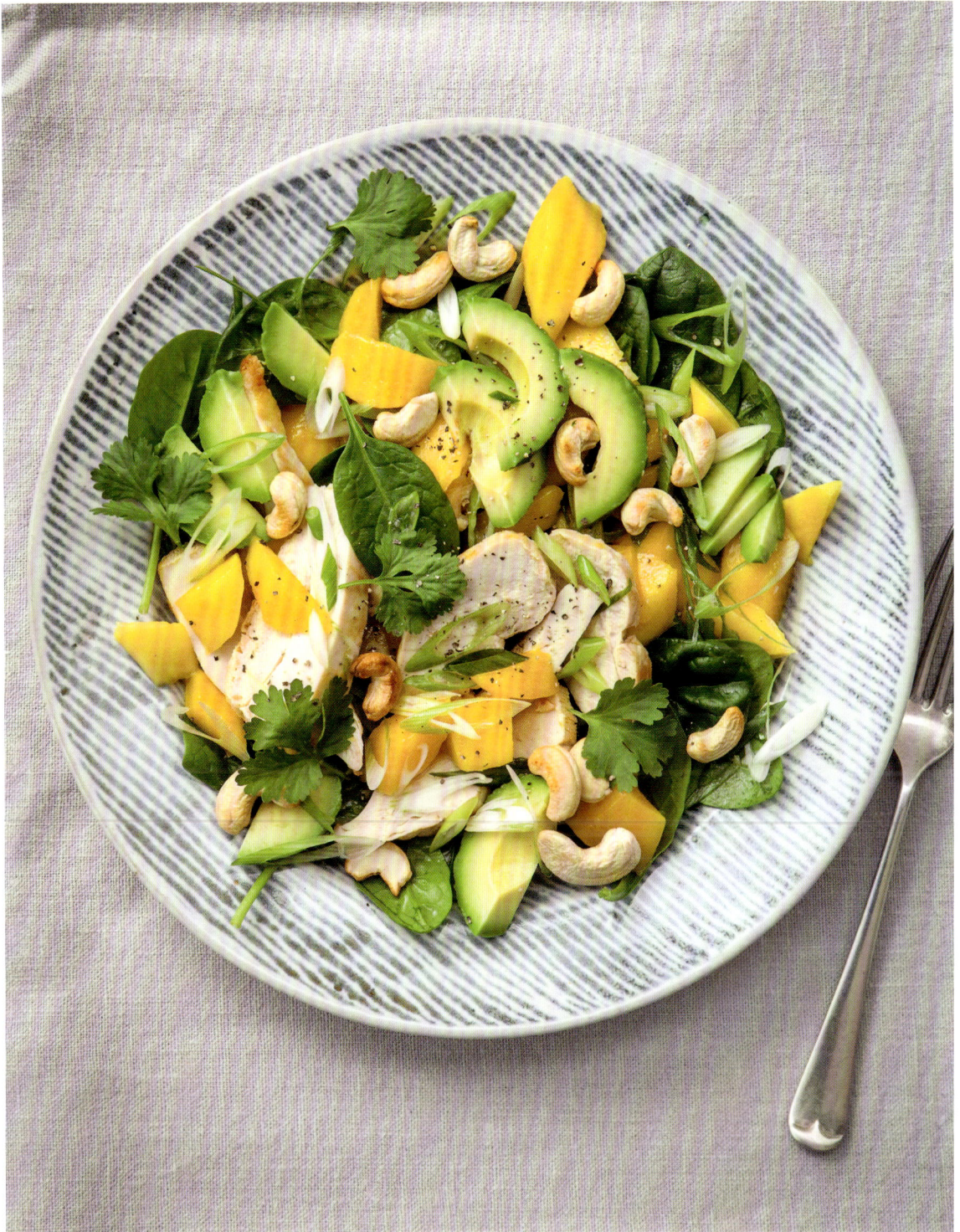

Steamed Pesto Salmon with Green Salad

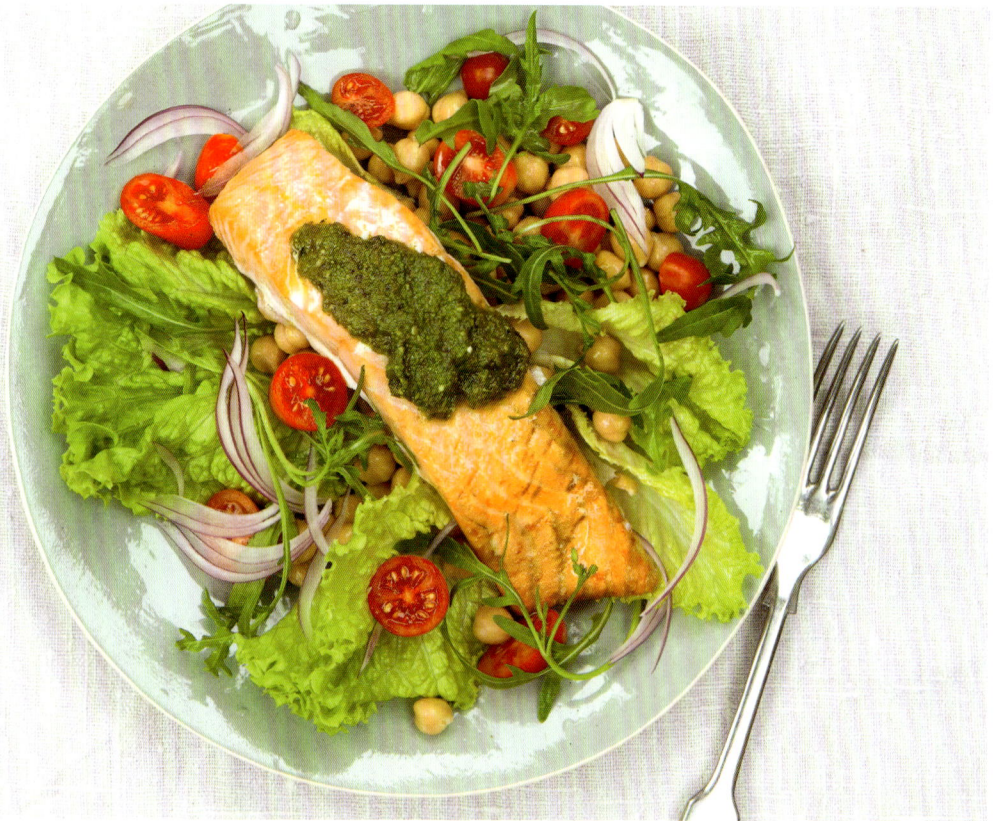

Serves 1

1 salmon fillet
1 tablespoon green pesto

To serve:
lettuce
handful of rocket
6 cherry tomatoes, halved
200g (7oz) canned chickpeas,
    drained and rinsed
½ red onion, thinly sliced

This delicious salad is nutrient-dense and quick to make. Red onions contain chromium, a mineral that assists insulin in blood sugar control. Balanced blood sugar levels are essential to help prevent those pesky sugar cravings.

1. Cook the salmon in a steamer over a saucepan of gently simmering water for 5–7 minutes until done to your liking. Alternatively, grill the salmon under a preheated hot grill for 12 minutes, turning once. Spoon the pesto over the salmon and serve on a bed of lettuce, rocket, cherry tomatoes, chickpeas and sliced red onion.

Chicken & Avocado Cabbage Wraps

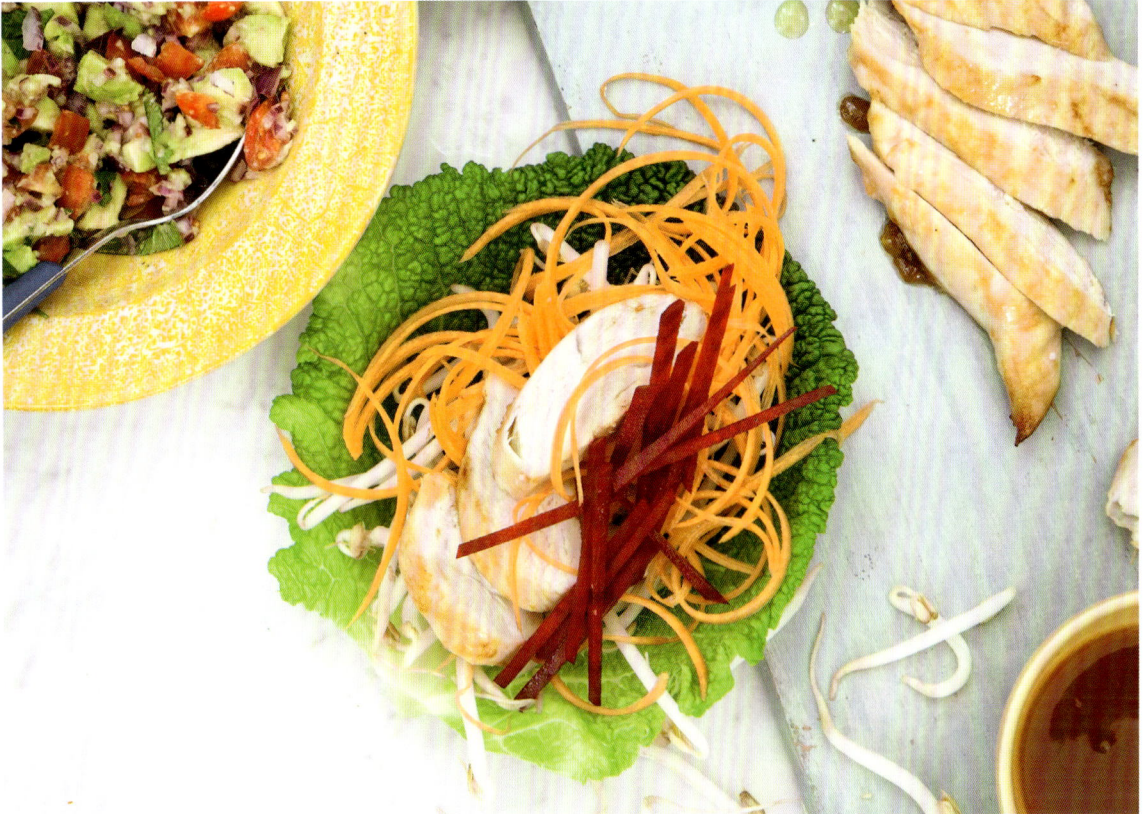

baby cabbage leaves
1 cooked chicken breast, sliced
½ avocado, chopped, or homemade salsa
   (see below)
handful of beansprouts
1 carrot, peeled and grated
1 small raw beetroot, peeled and grated
lemon or lime juice, for squeezing
Tabasco sauce, to taste

For homemade salsa:
1 large tomato, diced
½ red chilli, finely chopped
1 tablespoon chopped coriander
1 tablespoon lime juice
1 avocado, chopped
salt and black pepper

These wraps use cabbage rather than bread, which means they are higher in nutrients such as magnesium, vitamin K and fibre. They are also much easier on the digestive tract and don't make you feel sluggish.

1. If you are making your own salsa, mix all the salsa ingredients together in a small bowl and season well.

2. Lay out a few baby cabbage leaves and top with the chicken, avocado or salsa, beansprouts, carrot and beetroot.

3. Squeeze over some lemon or lime juice and add a dash of Tabasco sauce for a kick. Roll up and enjoy.

Courgette Fritters with Smoked Salmon

This delicious dish is perfect for breakfast or lunch, and is super simple to make. Courgettes are a good source of B vitamins, particularly folate, B2 and B6 – all of which are required for energy production in the body.

Serves 1

1 courgette, grated
1 egg
50g (1¾oz) gluten-free flour
1 tablespoon grated Parmesan
   cheese (optional)
olive oil, for frying
small handful of rocket
smoked salmon slices or trimmings
lemon juice, for squeezing
salt and black pepper

1. Place the grated courgette in a colander and sprinkle with a good pinch of salt. Leave to drain as long as you can – the longer you leave it, the crispier (and easier to cook) your fritters will be.

2. Squeeze the excess water out of the courgette, then place in a bowl with the egg, flour and Parmesan, if using. Season with a little salt and lots of pepper and stir well to combine.

3. Heat the oil in a frying pan. While it's warming, make the fritters by rolling the courgette mixture into little balls, then squishing them flat with your thumb. Place in the hot pan and cook for 1–2 minutes until golden underneath – a good way to tell if they're ready to turn is to give your pan a little shake; if they slide around easily, they're ready. Turn and cook for a further 1–2 minutes until golden on the other side, then transfer to a plate lined with kitchen paper to drain.

4. Pile the fritters on a plate with the rocket, top with the smoked salmon and finish with a good squeeze of lemon and a grinding of black pepper.

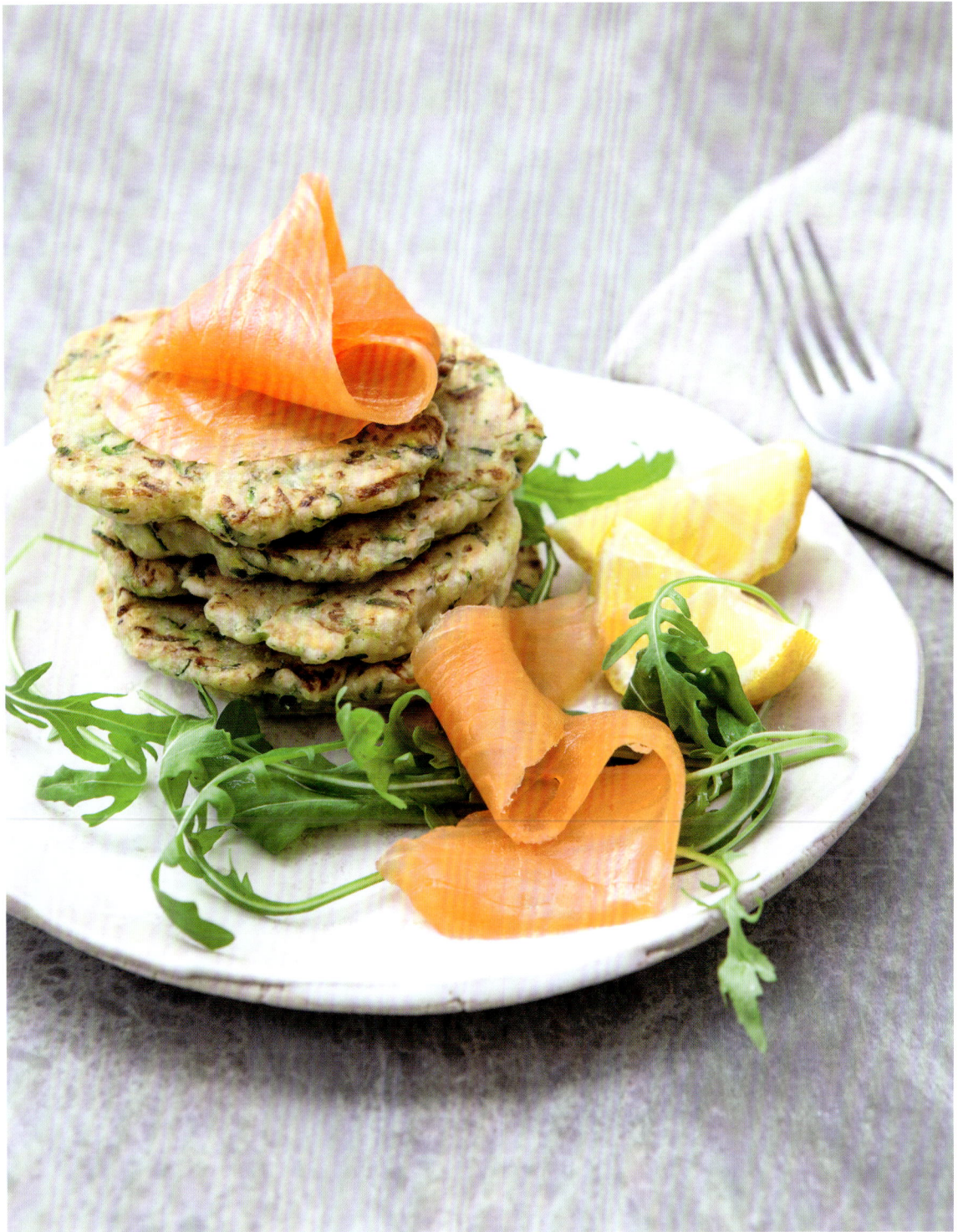

Spanish Omelette with Sweet Potato & Onion

This quick and simple recipe is the perfect ratio of carbs, fats and protein. It is a great option for when you are feeling super tired or are short on time.

<u>Serves 1</u>

2 eggs
1 teaspoon olive oil
1 onion, chopped
1 small sweet potato, cooked
   and diced
1 large tomato, diced
handful of feta cheese, diced
   (optional)
salt and black pepper

1. Beat the eggs in a small bowl and add a pinch of salt and pepper.

2. Heat the oil in a frying pan over a medium heat, add the onion and cook for 3–5 minutes, or until starting to soften. Add the sweet potato and cook for another 2 minutes, or until heated through.

3. Add the tomato and feta, if using, then pour over the eggs. Give everything a good stir then cook for about 5 minutes until the egg has set underneath. Transfer to a preheated hot grill and continue to cook for a further 1–2 minutes until the egg is set right through.

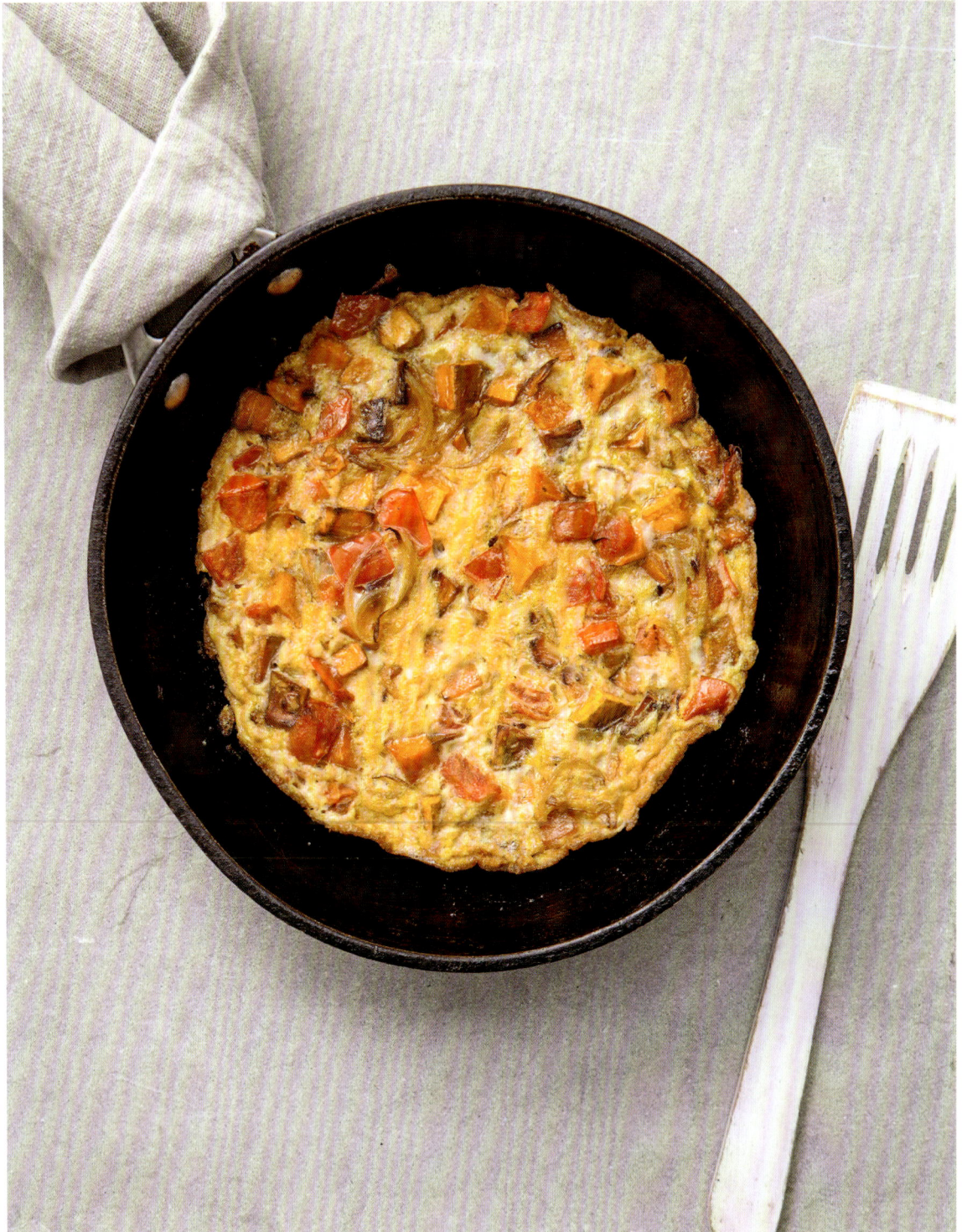

Avocado & Feta Pitta Pockets

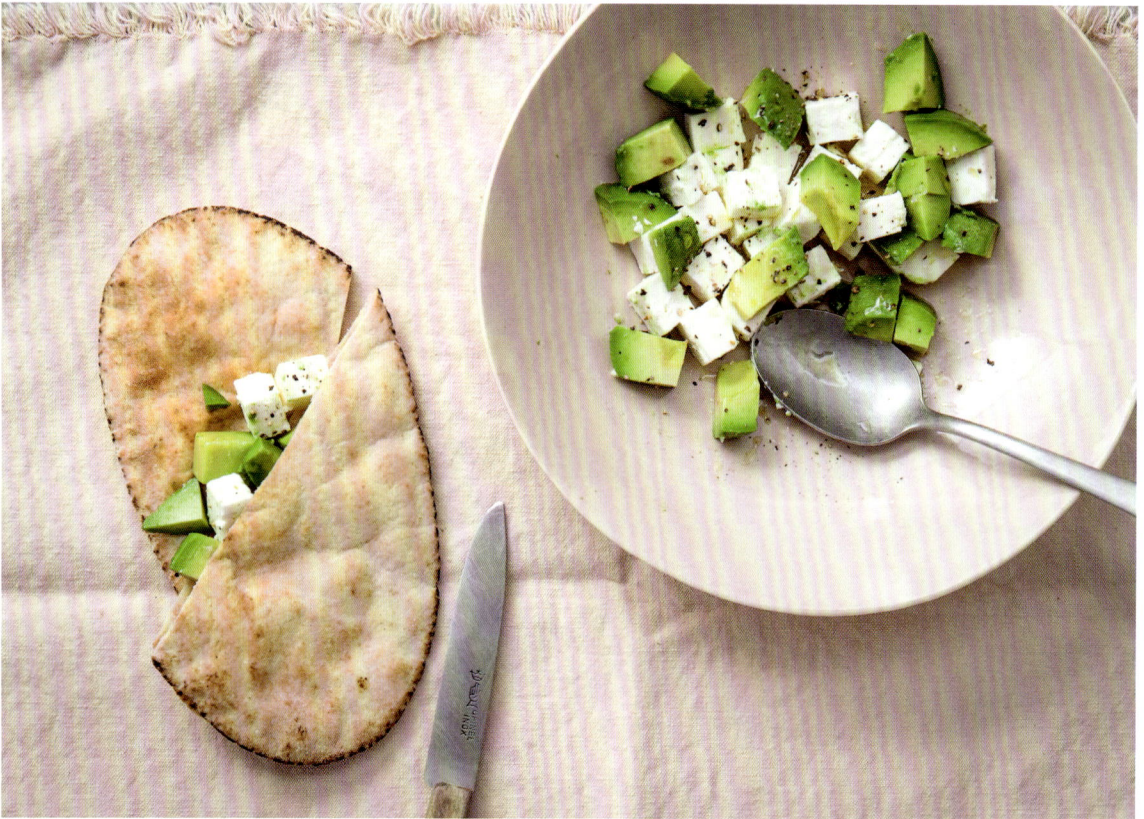

50g (1¾oz) feta cheese, diced
½ avocado, diced
olive oil, for drizzling
1 gluten-free pitta bread, toasted
black pepper

I love this lunch. It's tasty, satisfying and very fast to make. It's the perfect balanced meal if you're feeling exhausted.

1. Place the cheese and avocado in a bowl, drizzle with olive oil, season with pepper and toss together.

2. Halve the pitta bread and stuff the cheese mixture inside to make 2 pockets.

Lentil Dahl with Roasted Garlic

Serves 2

1 tablespoon butter or ghee

1 onion, chopped

2 green chillies, deseeded
and chopped

1 teaspoon finely chopped
fresh ginger

125g (4½oz) yellow or red lentils

850ml (1½ pints) water

3 tablespoons roasted garlic
purée or 4 garlic cloves,
crushed

1 teaspoon ground cumin

1 teaspoon ground coriander

200g (7oz) tomatoes, peeled
and diced

lemon juice, to taste

salt and black pepper

coriander leaves, chopped,
to serve

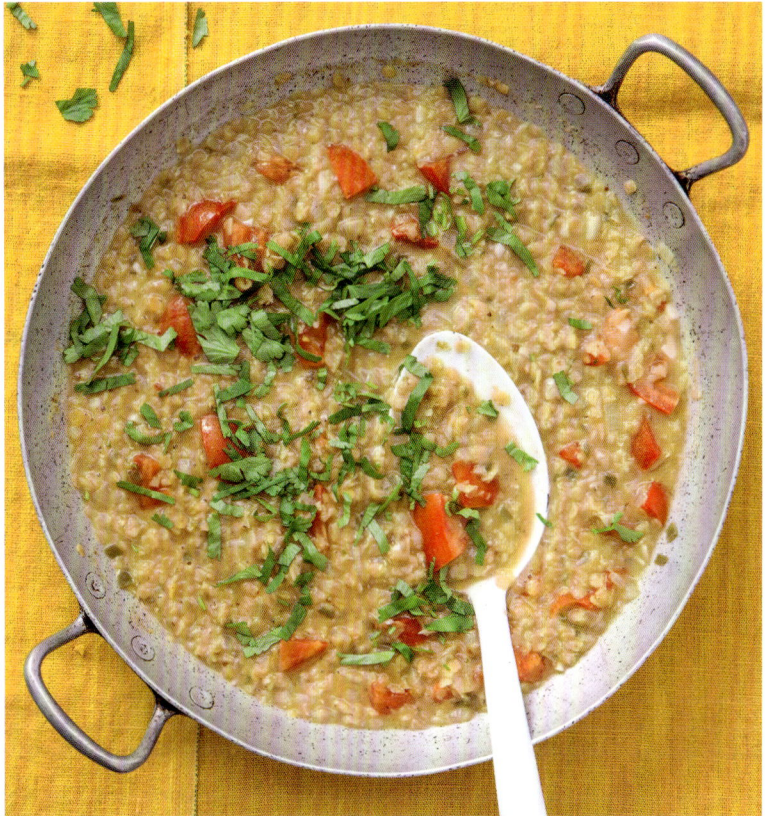

Lentils are an excellent source of protein, fibre, folate, iron, copper and zinc. They are comforting, warming and you can almost taste all those nutrients!

1. Melt the butter or ghee in a large saucepan over a medium heat, add the onion, chillies and ginger and cook for 10 minutes, stirring from time to time, until golden.

2. Stir in the lentils and measured water, bring to the boil then reduce the heat and partially cover the pan. Simmer, stirring occasionally, for 50–60 minutes until it is the consistency of a very thick soup.

3. Stir in the roasted garlic purée or crushed garlic, cumin and ground coriander, season to taste and cook for a further 10–15 minutes, uncovered, stirring frequently.

4. Stir in the tomatoes, adjust the seasoning and add lemon juice to taste. Serve topped with some chopped coriander leaves.

Garlic & Ginger Carrot Soup

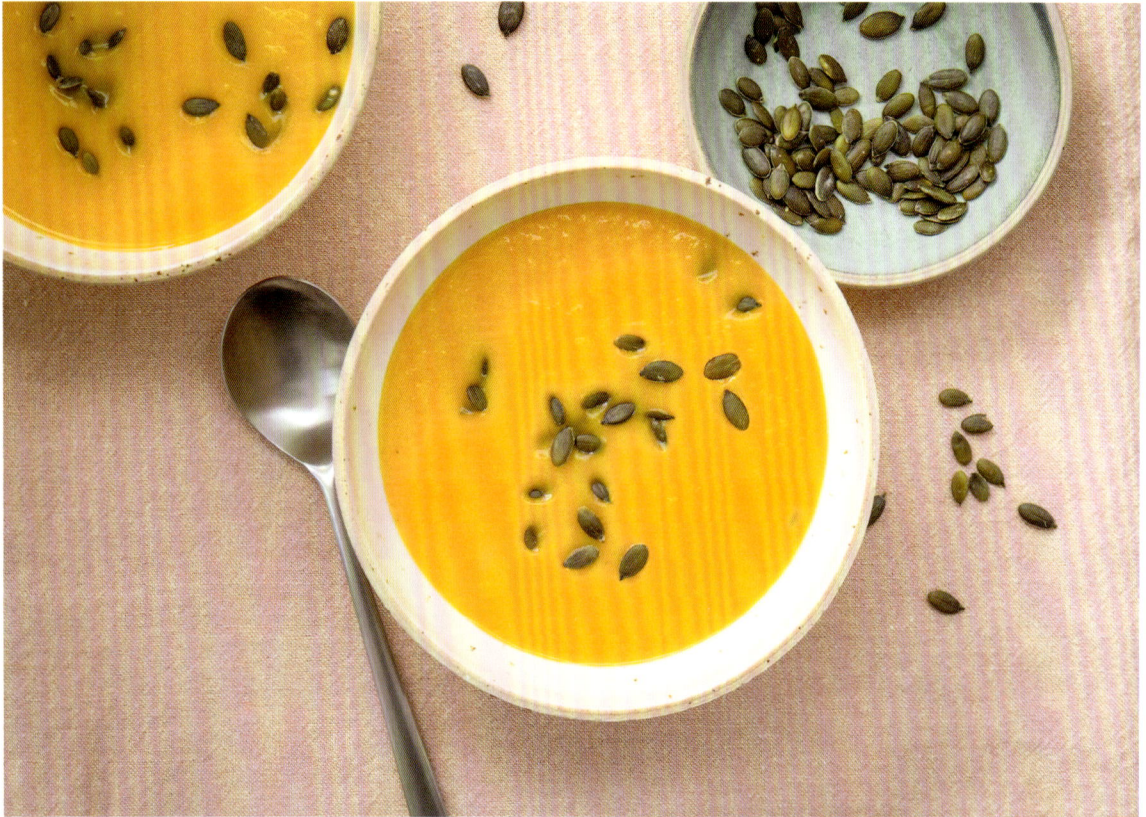

<u>Serves 4</u>

1 tablespoon olive oil
2 onions, chopped
2 garlic cloves, crushed
thumb-sized piece of fresh ginger,
    peeled and finely chopped
1 gluten-free stock cube
1 butternut squash, peeled, deseeded
    and cut into 2.5cm (1in) cubes
4 carrots, peeled and chopped
1.2 litres (2 pints) water
salt and black pepper
pumpkin seeds, to serve

This soup is super nourishing since it is a powerhouse of nutrients. Garlic and ginger help the immune system ward off germs or viruses that can make us feel run down and tired.

1. Heat the olive oil in a large saucepan over a medium heat, add the onions, garlic, ginger and stock cube and cook for 5 minutes, or until golden.

2. Add the squash and carrots and stir well, then add the water. Bring to the boil then reduce the heat and simmer for 20–30 minutes, or until the vegetables are soft. Remove from the heat, season to taste and blitz with a handheld blender until smooth. Serve sprinkled with pumpkin seeds.

Beetroot Soup

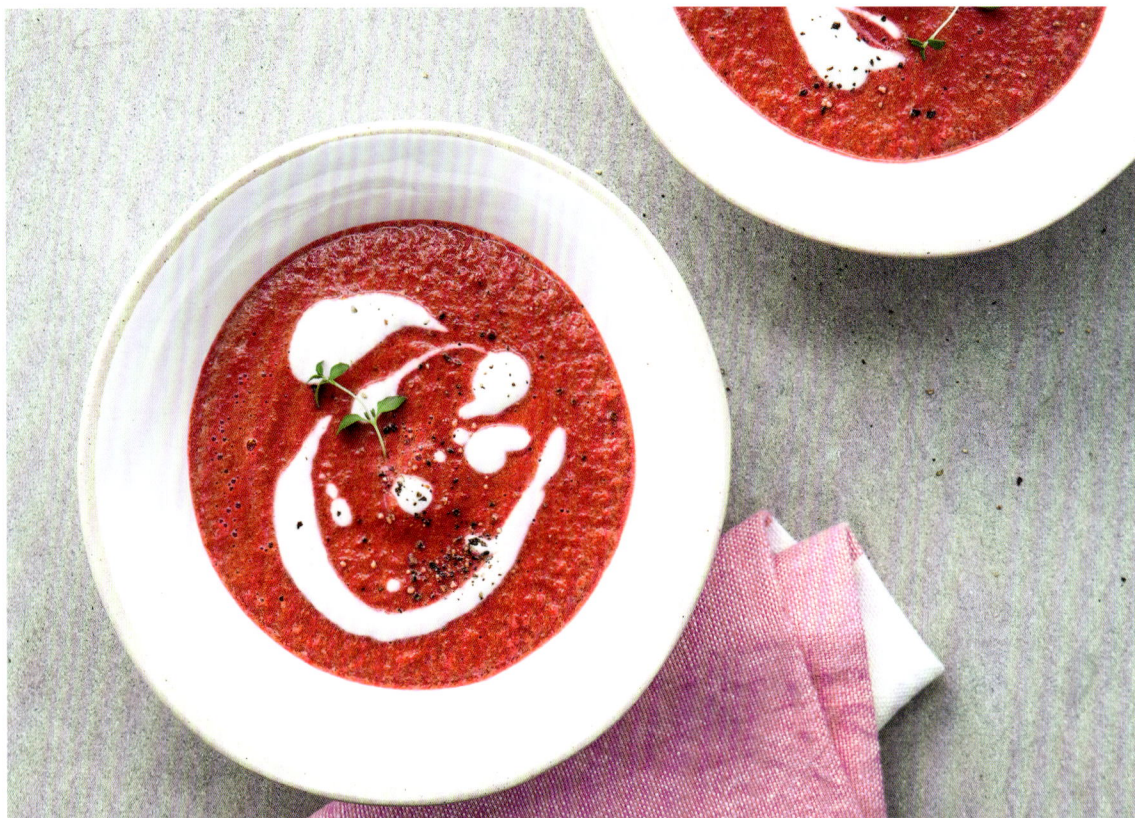

Serves 4

1 tablespoon olive oil
2 red onions, chopped
4 raw beetroots, diced
1 garlic clove, crushed
1 litre (1¾ pints) vegetable stock
3 tablespoons balsamic vinegar
handful of chopped thyme, plus
    extra to garnish
handful of chopped rosemary
200ml (7fl oz) coconut milk, plus
    extra to serve
salt and black pepper
gluten-free toast, to serve

Beetroot is one of my favourite foods. It is a great source of fibre, iron, potassium and vitamin C. Beetroot also helps to improve blood flow.

1. Heat the olive oil in a large saucepan over a medium heat, add the onions and cook for 3–5 minutes until softened. Add the beetroot and garlic and cook for a further 10 minutes, stirring often.

2. Add the stock, vinegar and herbs, bring to the boil then reduce the heat and simmer for an hour, or until the beetroot is soft.

3. Add the coconut milk, simmer gently for another 5 minutes, season to taste then remove from the heat. Blitz with a handheld blender until smooth, then serve in bowls with a swirl of coconut milk, a sprig of thyme and a grinding of black pepper. Serve with a slice of gluten-free toast.

Broccoli & Turmeric Soup

This nutritional soup is a delicious bowl of goodness. Turmeric has powerful anti-inflammatory properties. It improves blood flow and is effective in reducing pain in the body, particularly muscle pain and menstrual cramping.

Serves 2

1 tablespoon olive oil
1 onion, chopped
1 garlic clove, sliced
1 teaspoon ground turmeric
pinch of chilli flakes
1 small head of broccoli, roughly
    chopped
400g (14oz) can butter or cannellini
    beans, rinsed and drained
about 250ml (9fl oz) vegetable stock
salt and black pepper

1. Heat the olive oil in a large saucepan over a medium heat, add the onion and garlic and cook for 3–5 minutes until softened. Add the turmeric and chilli flakes and cook for a further 2 minutes.

2. Add the broccoli and beans, stir well, then add the stock – enough so that the broccoli and beans are covered. Bring to the boil then reduce the heat and simmer for about 8 minutes, or until the broccoli is cooked and soft. Remove from the heat and leave to rest for a minute or two. Blitz with a handheld blender to your desired consistency, then season to taste. Serve with an extra grinding of black pepper.

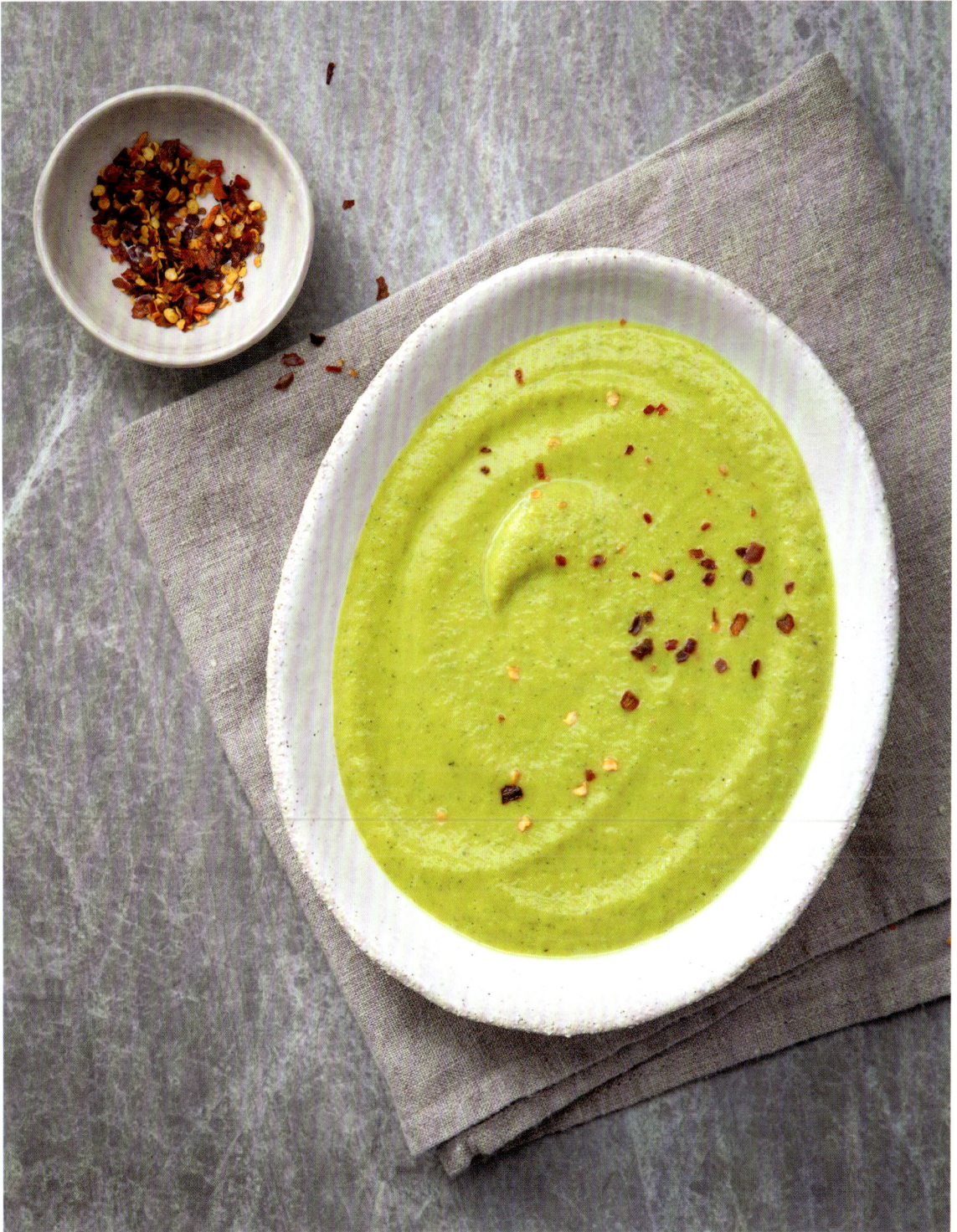

Coconut, Vegetable & Chicken Soup

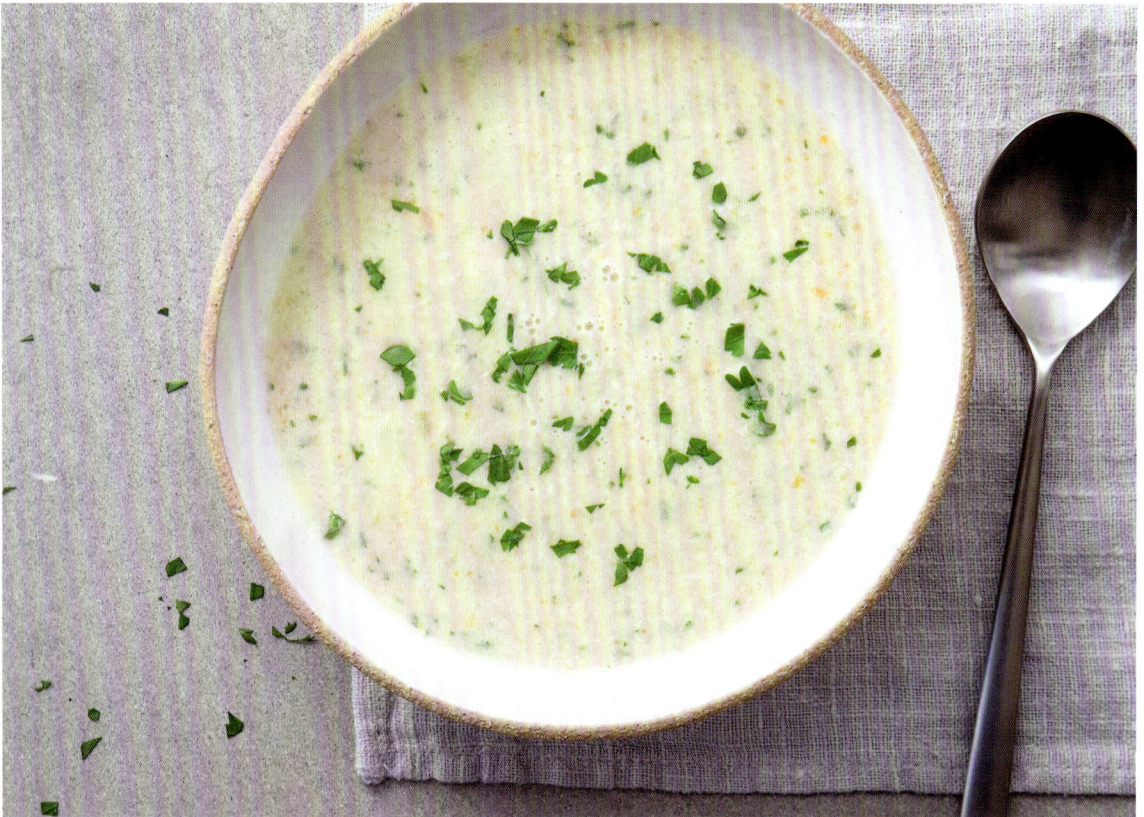

Serves 4

1 tablespoon olive oil
2 onions, chopped
1 garlic clove, crushed
2 celery sticks, chopped
1 gluten-free stock cube
100g (3½oz) chicken breast, chopped
2 carrots, peeled and chopped
1 litre (1¾ pints) water
200ml (7fl oz) coconut milk
handful of roughly chopped parsley,
    plus extra to garnish
salt and black pepper

I love using coconut milk in my cooking. It's got such a thick and creamy consistency, and because of the high fat content it's very energy dense.

1. Heat the oil in a large saucepan over a medium heat, add the onions, garlic and celery and cook for 5 minutes, or until soft and golden. Add the stock cube, chicken and carrots and cook for a further 10 minutes, or until the chicken turns white all over.

2. Pour in the water and coconut milk, bring to the boil then reduce the heat and simmer for 15 minutes.

3. Add the parsley, season to taste then remove from the heat. Blitz with a handheld blender until smooth, then serve garnished with extra parsley.

Roasted Tomato & Basil Soup

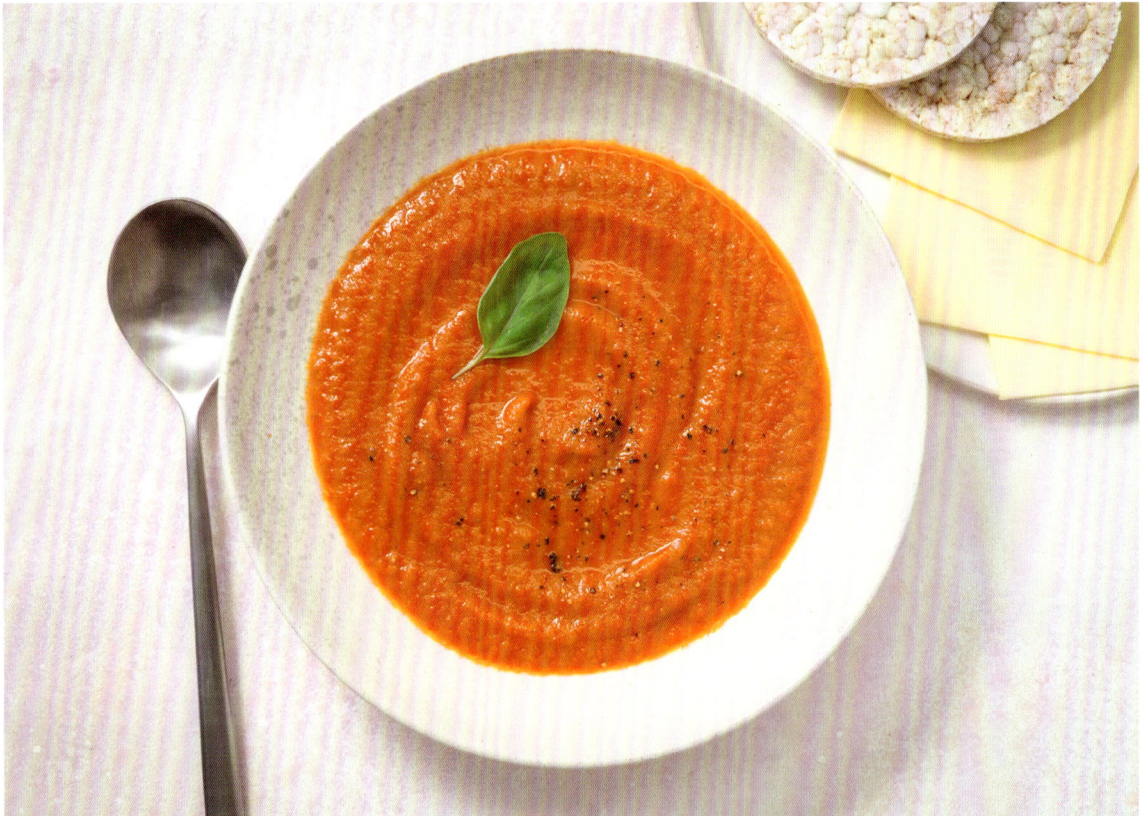

<u>Serves 2</u>

1 tablespoon olive oil
1 onion, chopped
2 garlic cloves, crushed
2 carrots, peeled and chopped
400g (14oz) can chopped tomatoes
500ml (18fl oz) vegetable stock
1 teaspoon balsamic vinegar
handful of basil leaves, plus extra
   to garnish
salt and black pepper
rice cakes and vegan cheese slices,
   to serve

This hearty soup is packed with antioxidants and nutrients. If you're hungry, enjoy it with rice cakes and vegan cheese slices, or two slices of gluten-free toast.

1. Heat the olive oil in a large saucepan over a medium heat, add the onion and garlic and cook for 3–5 minutes until softened.

2. Add the carrots, tomatoes, stock, vinegar and basil. Bring to the boil then reduce the heat and simmer for 30 minutes. Remove from the heat, season to taste and blitz with a handheld blender until smooth. Serve in bowls garnished with basil leaves, with two rice cakes and vegan cheese slices with each portion.

Dinner

Sweet Sea Bass Salad

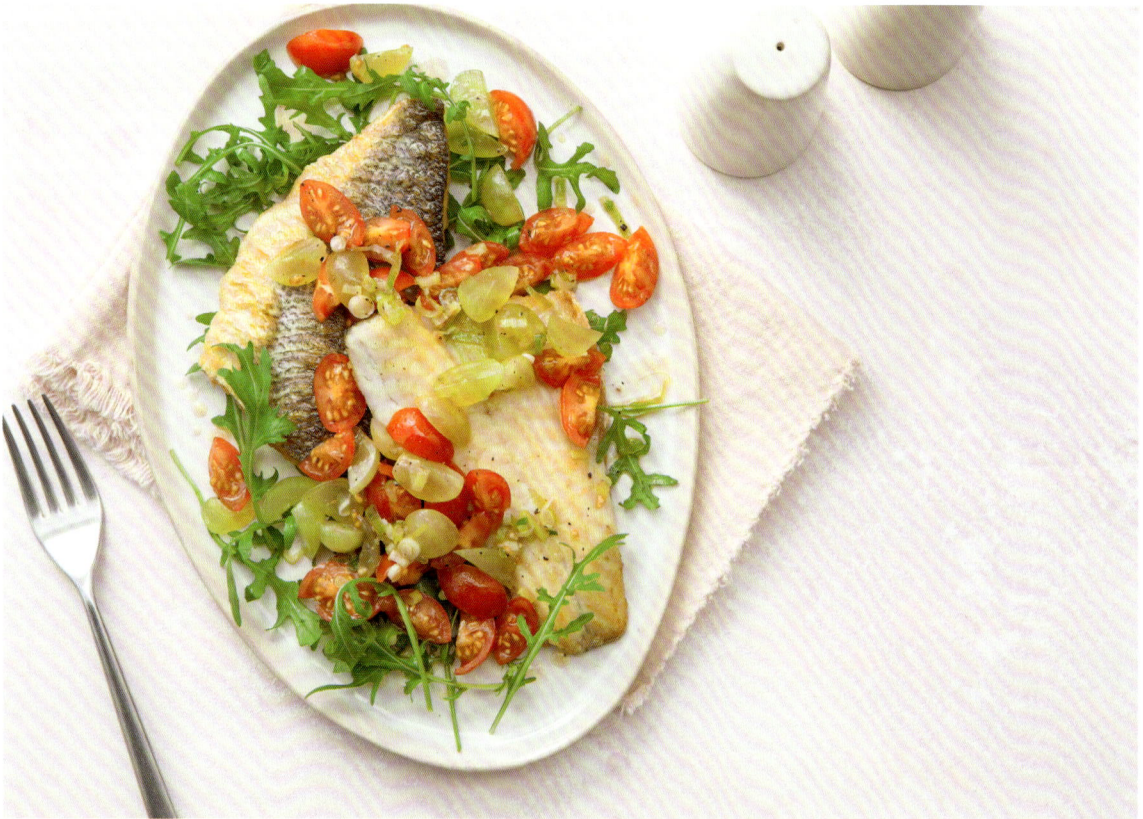

<u>Serves 1</u>

knob of butter
2 sea bass fillets
12 cherry tomatoes, chopped
12 large white grapes, chopped
1 spring onion, sliced
large handful of rocket
lemon juice, to taste
olive oil, for drizzling
salt and black pepper

This is probably one of the quickest dishes in the book and it is so good! Sea bass is a good source of iron, calcium and B12 as well as an excellent source of protein.

1. Melt the butter in a frying pan over a medium-high heat, add the bass fillets, skin side down, and cook for 3–5 minutes, or until the skin is crisp. Turn and cook for another minute, or until cooked through.

2. Place the tomatoes, grapes and spring onion in a bowl, squeeze over the lemon juice and drizzle with olive oil. Season to taste.

3. Arrange the rocket on a plate and top with the sea bass, followed by the tomato mixture. Drizzle over a little more oil and lemon juice and add a little more salt to taste.

Smoked Mackerel Layer Bake

Serves 2

1 smoked mackerel fillet, skinned
   and flaked
olive oil, for frying
1 garlic clove, sliced
large handful of spinach
1 raw beetroot, thinly sliced
1 large new potato, thinly sliced
1 egg
salt and black pepper
chopped chives, to garnish

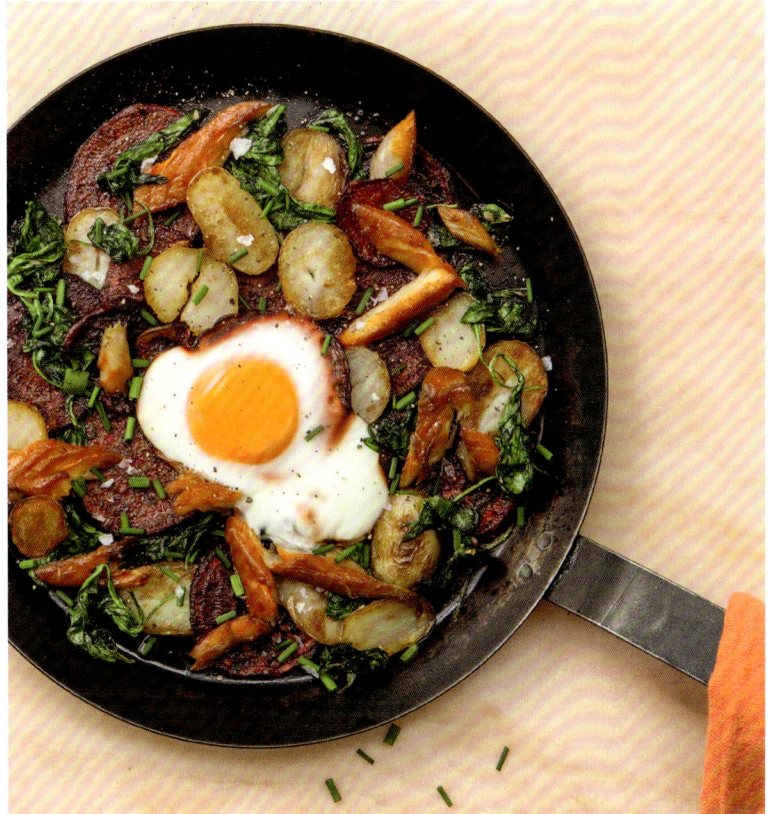

Mackerel is a rich source of omega-3 fatty acids. These are fundamental for brain and nerve function, including memory and concentration.

1. Preheat the oven to 190°C (375°F), Gas Mark 5. Arrange the flaked mackerel across the bottom of a small ovenproof dish. Heat a dash of olive oil in a large frying pan over a medium heat, add the garlic and cook for 1 minute, stirring, then add the spinach and cook until it just wilts but is still bright green. Season lightly and arrange over the top of the mackerel.

2. Heat a little more oil in the same frying pan, add the beetroot and potato slices and fry for around 5 minutes on both sides until golden brown and cooked through, cooking in batches if necessary. Layer the beetroot and potato over the spinach. Crack the egg on top, season well and bake in the oven for 10–15 minutes, or until the egg white is set but the yolk is still runny. Sprinkle over the chives and serve piping hot.

Prawn & Cashew Stir-fry

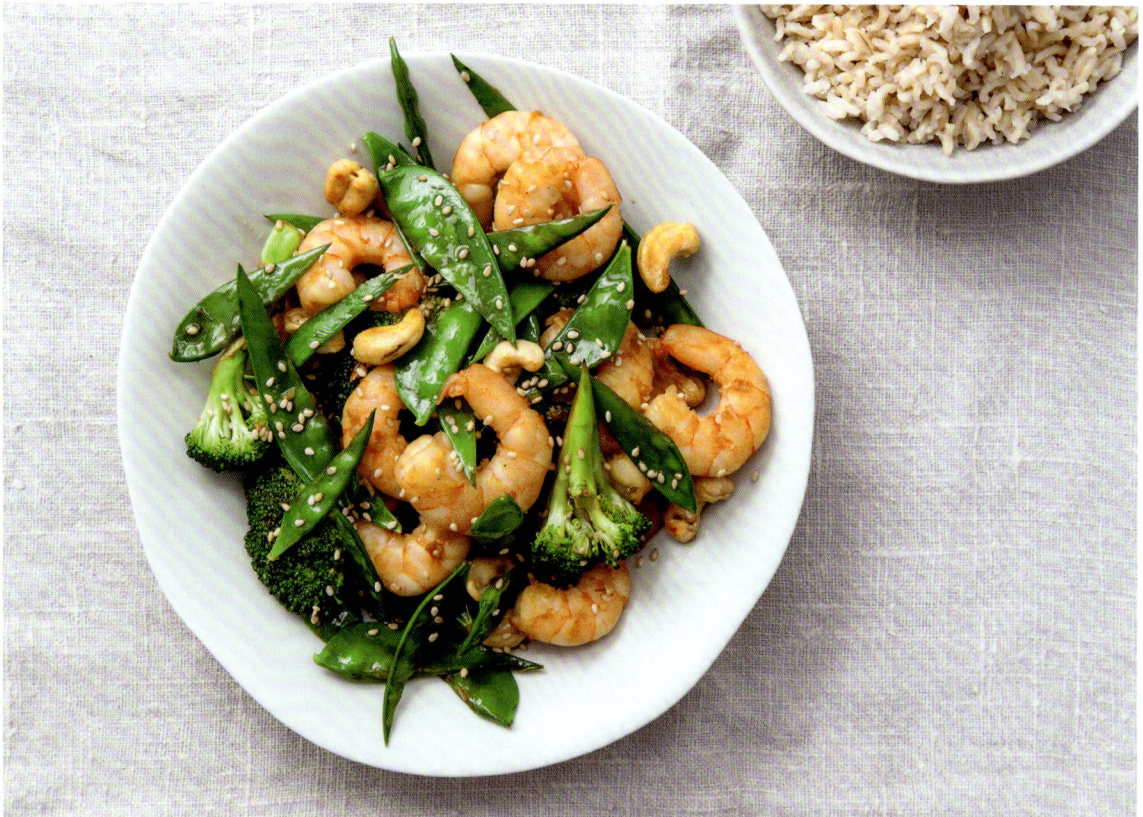

1 tablespoon sunflower oil
1 teaspoon sesame oil
150g (5½oz) cooked peeled
    king prawns
handful of broccoli florets
handful of mangetout
handful of cashew nuts
2 tablespoons sesame seeds
1 garlic clove, crushed
3 tablespoons soy sauce
brown rice, to serve

Cashew nuts are by far my favourite nut because they have a delicious creamy consistency. They also contain high levels of iron, magnesium, zinc, copper, phosphorus and manganese, so they are rich in nutrients.

1. Heat the two oils in a wok or frying pan over a high heat and add all the remaining ingredients. Cook, stirring regularly, for about 15 minutes, or until the veggies are tender, turning down the heat a little or adding a dash of water if it starts to catch. Serve with brown rice.

Puttanesca Prawn Pasta

Serves 4

1 tablespoon olive oil
1 red onion, diced
2 garlic cloves, sliced
pinch of dried chilli flakes
2 teaspoons tomato purée
2 canned anchovy fillets in
  olive oil
400g (14oz) can chopped
  tomatoes
1 tablespoon capers, drained
dash of red wine vinegar
75g (2¾oz) gluten-free
  spaghetti
150g (5½oz) cooked peeled
  king prawns
small handful of basil leaves
salt and black pepper

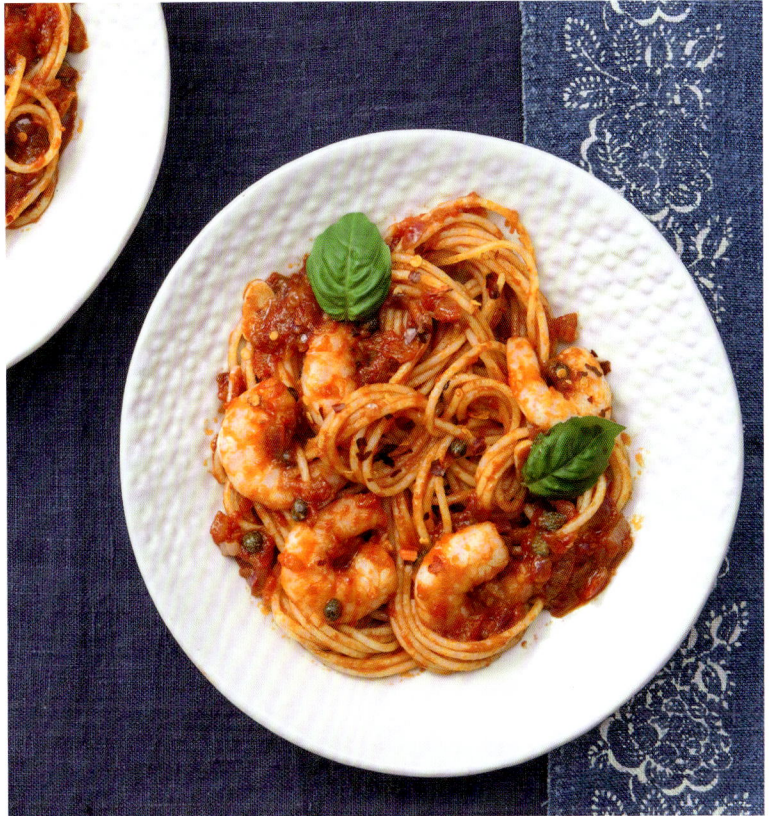

This dish is simple but classic. Did you know that 100g (3½ oz) of prawns provide 25g (1 oz) of protein? They are also a rich source of selenium, phosphorus and vitamin E.

1. Heat the olive oil in a saucepan over a medium heat, add the onion and garlic and cook for 5 minutes, or until softened. Add the chilli flakes, tomato purée and anchovies and cook, stirring, until the anchovies have melted into the oil.

2. Add the tomatoes, capers and a dash of red wine vinegar, bring to the boil, then lower the heat and leave to simmer and thicken while you cook the pasta.

3. Cook the spaghetti in a saucepan of lightly salted boiling water according to packet instructions, then drain well and add to the sauce along with the prawns. Season to taste and mix well over the heat so that the prawns warm through. Serve immediately, scattered with the basil leaves.

Baked Salmon with Butter Bean Mash

Butter beans are great in plant-based dishes because they have a meaty texture and are very filling. They are a fab source of B vitamins, which are essential for converting carbohydrates into energy.

Serves 1

1 salmon fillet
1 teaspoon olive oil
lemon juice, for drizzling
knob of butter
2 garlic cloves, crushed
1 red onion, sliced
1 tablespoon balsamic vinegar
1 tablespoon honey
salt and black pepper
lemon wedges, to serve

Butter bean mash
400g (14oz) can butter beans, rinsed and drained
juice of ½ lemon
handful of chopped chives
handful of chopped parsley
1 tablespoon olive oil

1. Preheat the oven to 200°C (400°F), Gas Mark 6. Place the salmon on a square of foil large enough to wrap it completely. Drizzle with the olive oil and some lemon juice, season to taste and bring the edges of the foil together, folding them over to make an airtight parcel. Place on a baking tray and cook for 20–25 minutes, or until cooked to your liking.

2. Meanwhile, melt the butter in a small saucepan over a medium-low heat, add the garlic, onion, vinegar and honey and cook for 5–7 minutes until caramelized and soft, reducing the heat if it starts to catch. Remove from the heat and set aside.

3. For the butter bean mash, place all the ingredients in a food processor, season to taste and blitz until smooth and fluffy. Transfer to a saucepan and heat over a low-medium heat for 5 minutes until hot.

4. Transfer the mash to a plate, pile the onions on top and serve with the salmon and lemon wedges for squeezing. Eat immediately.

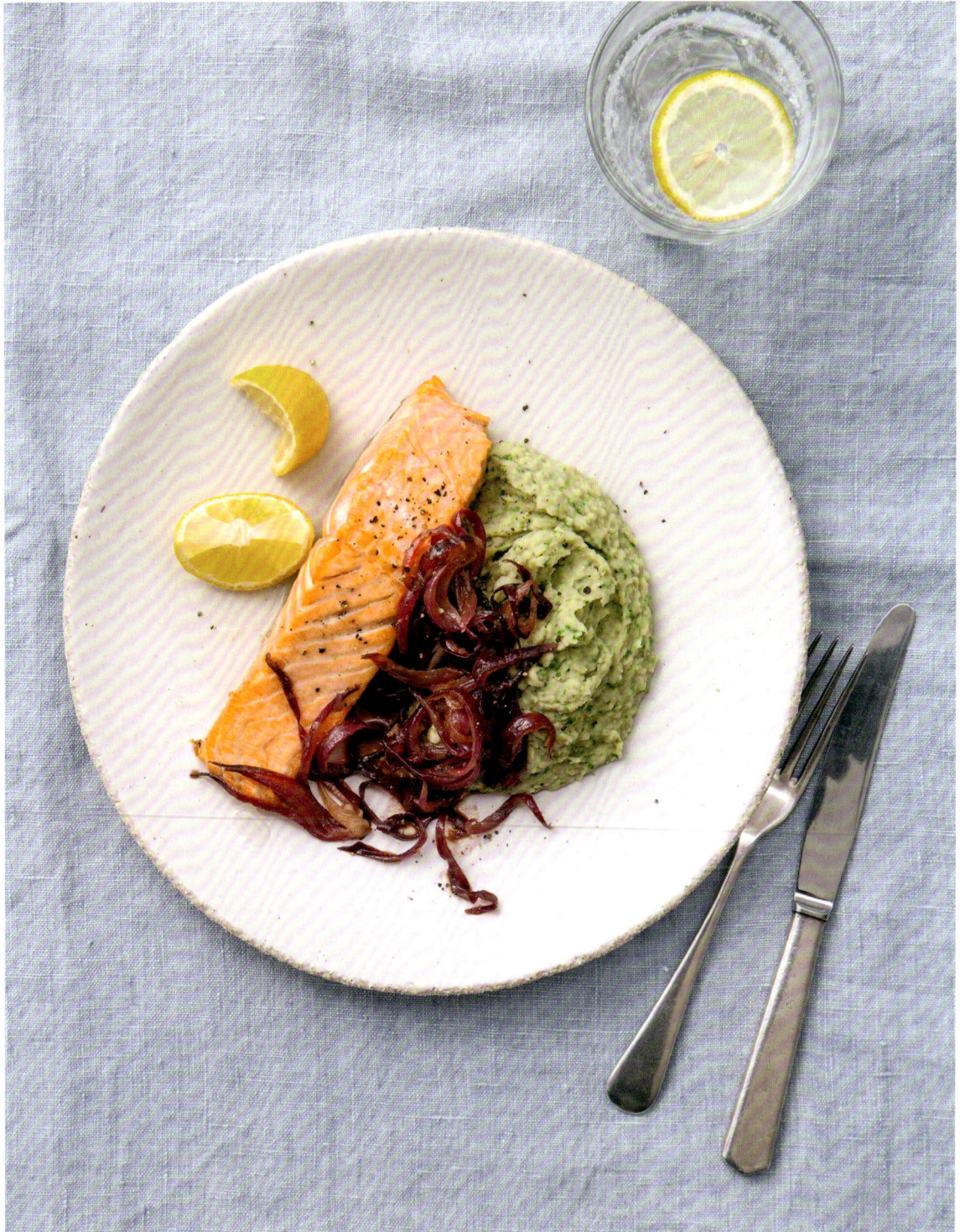

Steamed Ginger & Soy Fish Parcels

180g (6½oz) wild rice
2 sustainable white fish fillets
2 thumb-sized pieces of fresh
    ginger, peeled and cut into
    matchsticks
1 red chilli, thinly sliced
2 spring onions, thinly sliced
4 teaspoons sesame oil
4 teaspoons rice wine vinegar
4 teaspoons soy sauce
juice of 1 lime
2 teaspoons honey
black pepper
leafy green vegetables, to serve

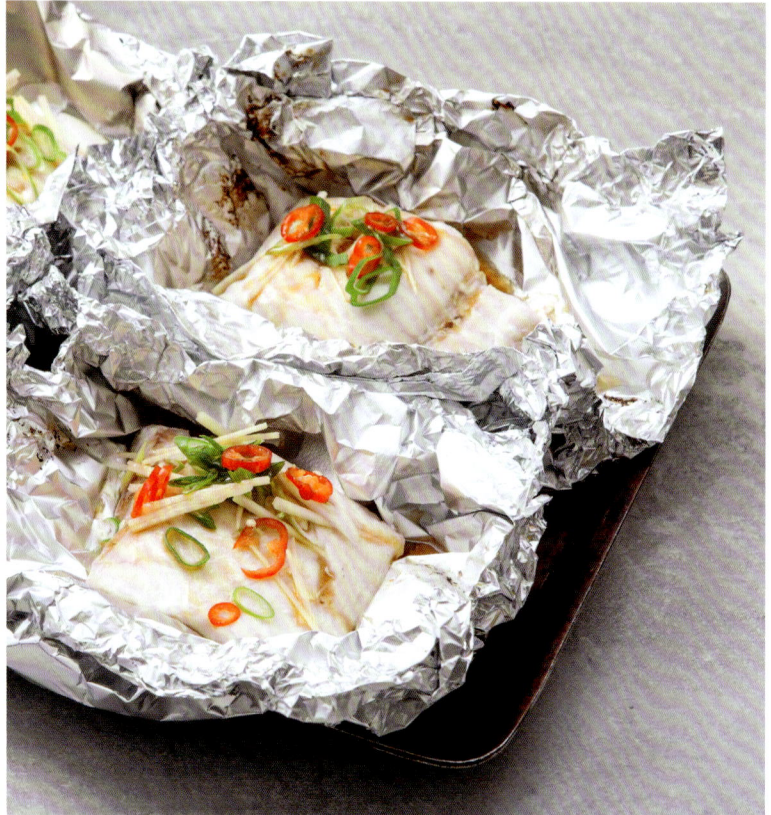

Ginger is excellent for calming the gut, helping to reduce nausea, gas and bloating. Grate it onto your food or add to some hot water and drink with a squeeze of honey.

1. Preheat the oven to 190°C (375°F), Gas Mark 5. Cook the wild rice in a saucepan of lightly salted boiling water according to packet instructions. Drain and keep warm.

2. Meanwhile, place each fish fillet on a square of foil large enough to wrap it completely and top each with half of the ginger, chilli and spring onions.

3. Mix the sesame oil, rice wine vinegar, soy sauce, lime juice and honey in small bowl. Bring up the edges of the foil around the fish fillets and pour three-quarters of the sauce over both.

4. Season with pepper and bring the edges of the foil together, folding them over to make an airtight parcel for each fillet. Place on a baking tray and cook for 10–15 minutes, or until cooked to your liking.

5. Open the parcels, pour over the remaining sauce and serve on two plates with the wild rice and some leafy green veggies.

Pan-fried Cod with Mint Pea Mash

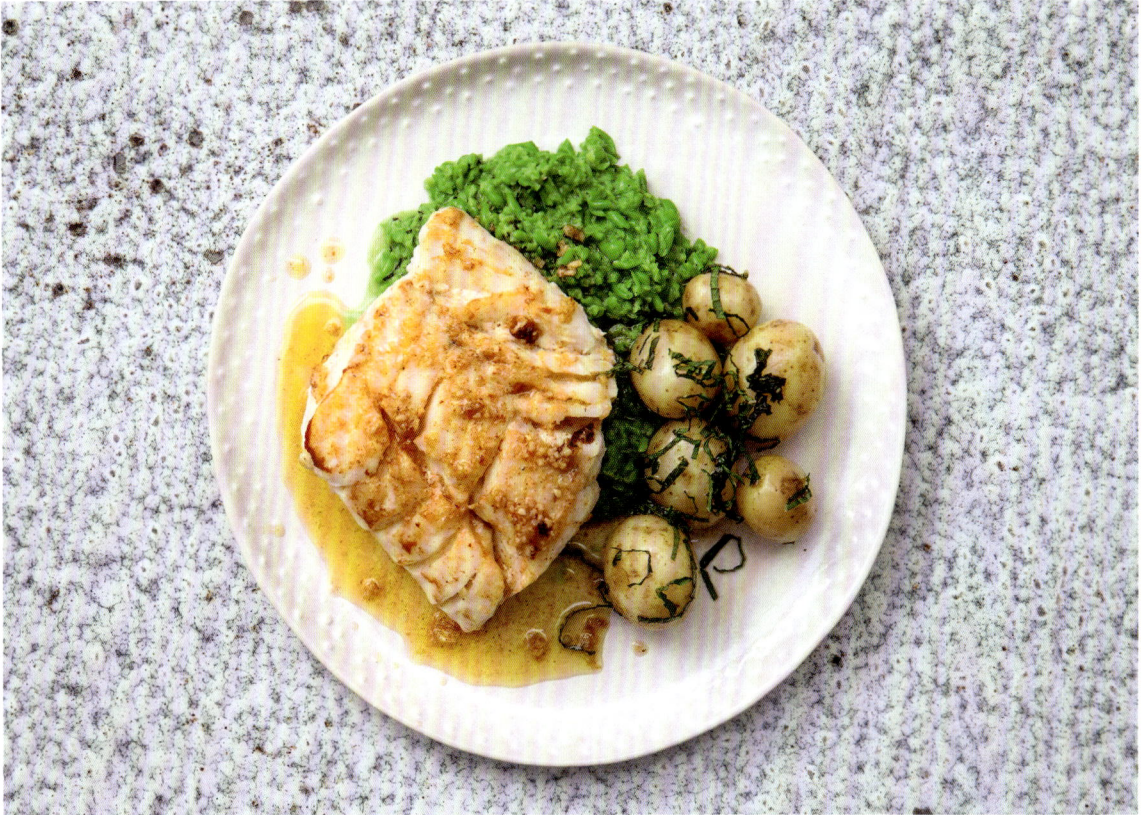

Serves 1

1 tablespoon olive oil
1 garlic clove, crushed
1 cod fillet
50g (1¾oz) frozen peas, defrosted
2 mint sprigs, leaves picked
200ml (7fl oz) coconut milk
salt and black pepper
new potatoes, to serve

Cod is a great source of B12, which is a co-factor for ATP, your body's energy source. It also doesn't take long to cook and is a reliable source of protein.

1. Heat the oil in a frying pan over a medium heat, add the garlic and lay the cod on top. Season to taste and cook for about 3 minutes on each side until cooked through and golden.

2. Meanwhile, place the peas, mint leaves and coconut milk in a food processor, season to taste and blitz until smooth. Transfer to a saucepan and heat over a medium-low heat for 5 minutes, or until hot.

3. Spoon the pea mixture onto a plate and place the cod on top. Serve with new potatoes.

Grilled Fish Kebabs

I love this dish! You can use any fish or vegetables you have to hand but I've included salmon here because it's an excellent source of essential fats.

<u>Serves 2</u>

200g (7oz) salmon or monkfish, cubed
10 cooked peeled king prawns
1 yellow pepper, cored, deseeded and cut into chunks
1 courgette, cut into chunks
2 red onions, cut into chunks
garlic oil, for drizzling
salt and black pepper

To serve:
sweet potato wedges
tartare sauce

1. Thread the fish, prawns and vegetables onto wooden or metal skewers – it doesn't matter which order they go in. Arrange on a baking tray lined with foil, drizzle with garlic oil and season to taste.

2. Cook the kebabs under a preheated medium-high grill, turning from time to time, for about 10 minutes, or until cooked through. Serve with sweet potato wedges and small servings of tartare sauce.

YOUR NEW FOOD MANTRA:

'If it didn't come from the ground,
or didn't have a mother...

Don't eat it!'

Stick to natural foods wherever possible.
You'll soon feel the benefits.

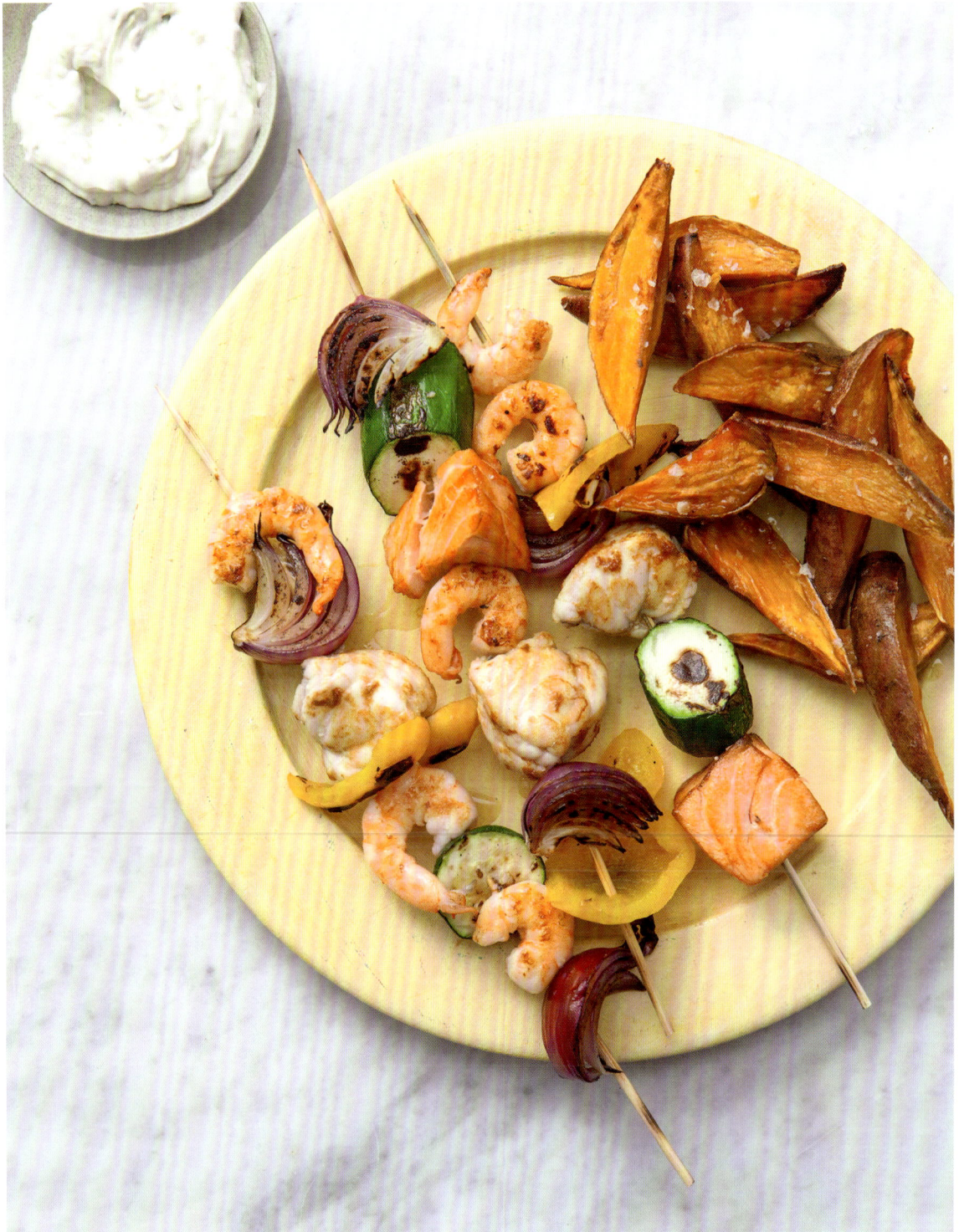

Salmon Fishcakes

400g (14oz) salmon fillet
450g (1lb) sweet potatoes, diced
finely grated zest and juice of
   1 lemon
2 spring onions, finely sliced
1 garlic clove, crushed
1 small red chilli, finely chopped
1 heaped teaspoon wholegrain
   mustard
small handful of chopped
   parsley
1 tablespoon olive oil, plus extra
   for frying
1–2 eggs, beaten
2 tablespoons rice flour
salt and black pepper
green salad, to serve

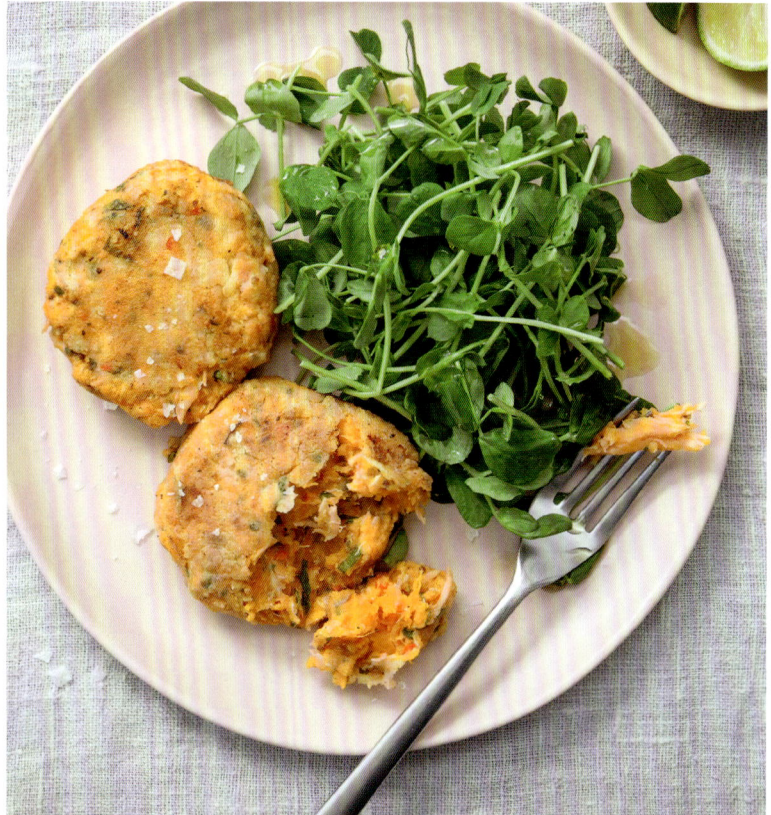

These fishcakes are delicious. If you're not going to eat them all in one go, freeze them uncooked for a later date.

1. Preheat the oven to 180°C (350°F), Gas Mark 4. Place the salmon on a baking tray and cook for 12–15 minutes, or until just cooked through. Remove from the oven and leave until cool enough to handle, then flake the flesh, removing any skin and bones.

2. Meanwhile, cook the sweet potatoes in a saucepan of lightly salted boiling water for 10–15 minutes, or until tender. Drain well and mash until smooth.

3. Place the salmon and sweet potato in a large bowl and add the lemon zest and juice, spring onions, garlic, chilli, mustard, parsley and olive oil. Season to taste and gently combine the ingredients together, without breaking up the fish too much.

4. Using damp hands, form the mixture into 8 equal-sized balls, then flatten into patty shapes. Chill in the refrigerator for 10–15 minutes, to firm up. If you aren't planning to cook all the fishcakes at once, they can be frozen at this stage.

5. Place the egg and flour in separate shallow bowls. Dip the fishcakes first in the egg and then the flour, to coat evenly all over. Heat a little olive oil in a large frying pan over a medium-high heat and cook the fishcakes for a few minutes until golden brown on each side. Serve with a green salad.

Quick Fish Stew with Olives & Lemon

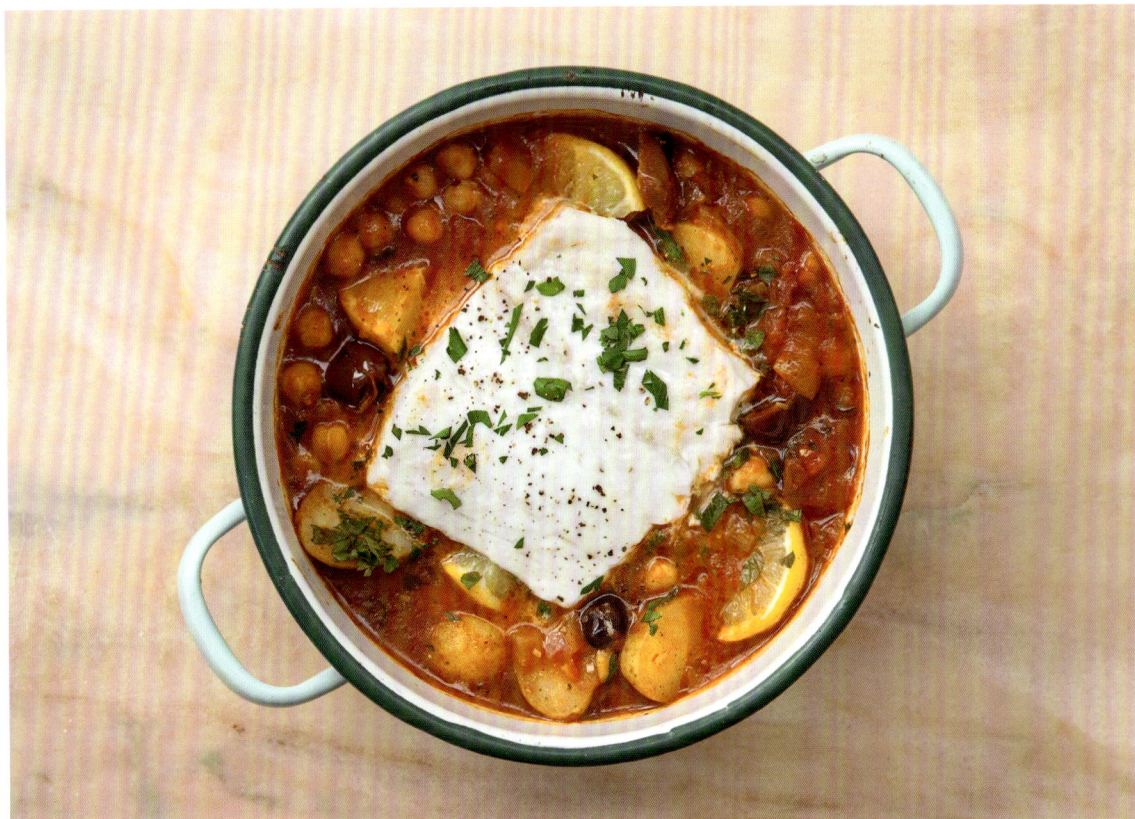

1 tablespoon olive oil

1 onion, diced

2 garlic cloves, sliced

2 canned anchovy fillets in olive oil

1 gluten-free vegetable stock cube

400g (14oz) can chopped tomatoes

400g (14oz) can chickpeas, drained
   and rinsed

handful of Kalamata olives, pitted
   and roughly chopped

handful of new potatoes, halved

handful of chopped flat leaf parsley

1 lemon, quartered

1 chunky sustainable white fish fillet,
   such as cod, sea bream or monkfish

salt and black pepper

This hearty stew is a great source of protein, healthy fats and carbs. You can eat it warm or cold.

1. Heat the oil in a large casserole over a medium heat and add the onion, garlic and anchovies. Cook for 3–5 minutes until starting to soften. Add the stock cube and crush it into the pan, then add the tomatoes and bring to the boil.

2. Fill the empty tomato can with water and add to the pan, along with the chickpeas, olives and new potatoes. Bring to the boil again, then reduce the heat and simmer for 10 minutes, or until the potatoes are tender, adding a little more water if it becomes too dry. Stir in the parsley and lemon quarters and season well.

3. Lay the fish on top of the stew so that it's just submerged in the liquid but isn't pushed right to the bottom of the pan. Cover the pan and simmer gently for about 8 minutes, or until the fish is cooked through.

Roast Squash Quinoa Risotto

Serves 3-4

1 small butternut squash,
    peeled, deseeded and diced
2 tablespoons olive oil, plus
    extra to serve
1 tablespoon balsamic vinegar
small knob of butter (optional)
1 onion, diced
2 garlic cloves, sliced
1 teaspoon ground turmeric
100g (3½oz) risotto rice
75g (2¾oz) tricolour quinoa
500ml (18fl oz) hot vegetable
    stock
1 tablespoon coconut milk
splash of white wine (optional)
salt and black pepper
chopped flat leaf parsley,
    to garnish

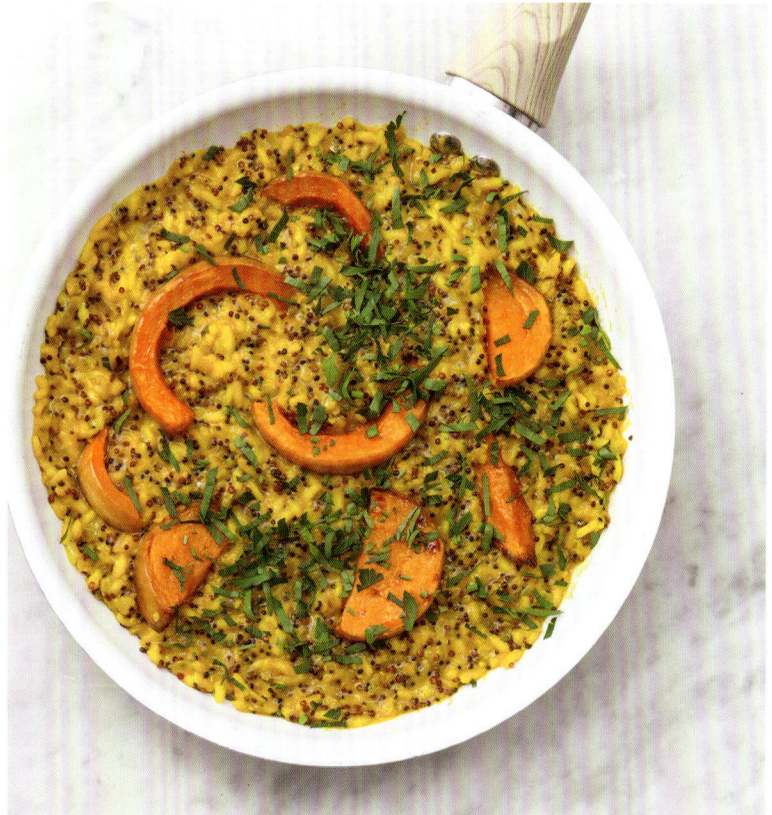

This dish is packed with slow-release carbohydrates to give you energy. I've used quinoa for protein, and butternut squash, which is a good source of vitamins A, B6 and C, folate and magnesium.

1. Preheat the oven to 190°C (375°F), Gas Mark 5. Place the squash on a baking tray, drizzle with half the oil and the balsamic vinegar, season to taste and toss together to coat the squash. Cook for about 25 minutes, or until golden brown.

2. Meanwhile, heat the remaining oil with the butter, if using, in a large saucepan over a medium heat and add the onion and garlic. Cook for 5 minutes, stirring often, until softened. Add the turmeric, rice and quinoa and stir well to coat in the onion mixture. Reserve a ladleful of hot stock for later, and then add a ladleful to the pan. Cook, stirring, until it has been absorbed. Add more stock and continue to cook and stir, adding more stock as it is absorbed.

3. Place half the butternut squash in a food processor with the reserved ladleful of hot stock and the coconut milk, season to taste and blitz until smooth. You're looking for a soup-like consistency. Add this to the risotto with the wine (if using) and the remaining squash. Stir well, check if the rice is cooked, and test the seasoning – you'll probably need a good pinch of both salt and pepper. Serve with an extra drizzle of olive oil and a sprinkle of chopped parsley.

Turkey & Aubergine Parmigiana

Serves 2

1 tablespoon olive oil, plus extra
    for brushing and drizzling
1 red onion, diced
1 garlic clove, sliced
400g (14oz) can chopped
    tomatoes
splash of red wine vinegar
1 aubergine, cut into 1cm (½in)
    slices
2 turkey steaks
1 ball of mozzarella, torn
handful of grated Parmesan
    cheese
salt and black pepper

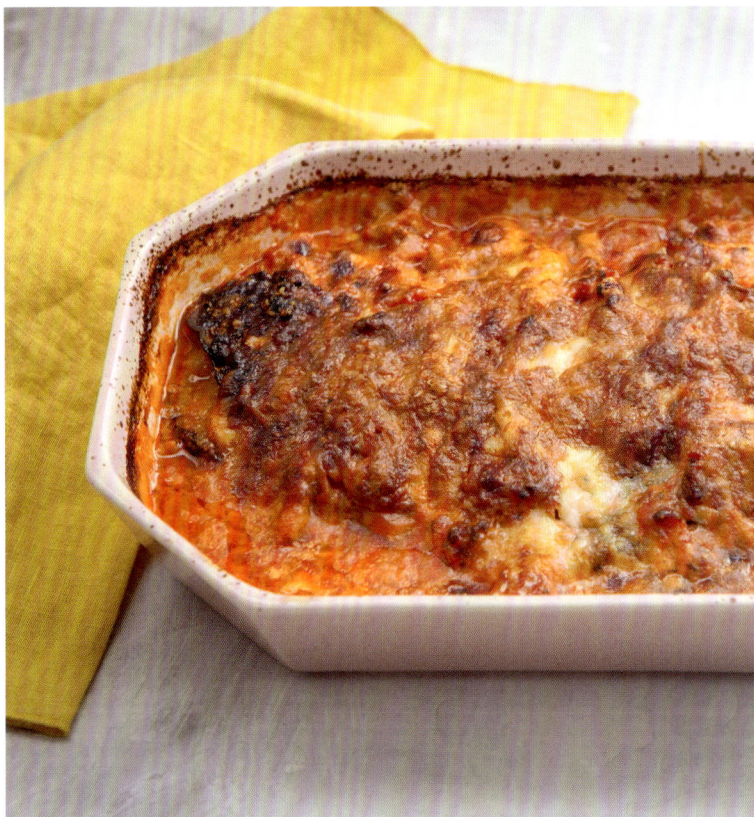

Aubergines are a great source of fibre and antioxidants. I find them delicious and very versatile.

1. Preheat the oven to 190°C (375°F), Gas Mark 5. Heat the oil in a saucepan over a medium heat, add the onion and garlic and cook for 5 minutes, or until softened. Add the tomatoes and vinegar and season to taste. Bring to the boil then reduce the heat and simmer for 15 minutes, or until nice and thick.

2. Meanwhile, brush the aubergine slices with olive oil, arrange in a single layer on a baking tray and season to taste. Cook for 15–20 minutes, or until golden and soft.

3. Spread half of the tomato sauce over the base of an ovenproof dish, then lay the turkey steaks on top. Arrange the aubergine slices over the top of the turkey, cover with half the mozzarella and season well. Top with the remaining tomato sauce, mozzarella and the Parmesan. Drizzle with a little olive oil and add a good grinding of black pepper. Cook for about 30 minutes, or until the turkey is cooked through and the cheese is golden and bubbling on top.

Avocado Pesto Spaghetti

Use gluten-free pasta in this dish to avoid an energy slump. You could also try replacing the spaghetti with any gluten-free grain such as brown rice or quinoa.

Serves 1

75g (2¾oz) gluten-free spaghetti
1 small avocado, pitted
handful of basil leaves
2 garlic cloves, roughly chopped
2 teaspoons pine nuts or cashew nuts
2 tablespoons olive oil
juice of 1 lemon
salt and black pepper
grated Parmesan, to serve (optional)

1. Cook the spaghetti in a saucepan of lightly salted boiling water according to packet instructions.

2. Meanwhile, place the avocado, basil, garlic and pine nuts in a food processor and season to taste. Blitz to combine. With the processor running on a low setting, slowly and steadily pour in the olive oil and lemon juice and blend until creamy – you may need to add a little of the pasta cooking water to loosen it.

3. Drain the spaghetti, retaining a spoonful or two of the cooking water, and mix well with the pesto, adding the water if necessary to loosen it. Serve with grated Parmesan, if using, and a good grinding of black pepper.

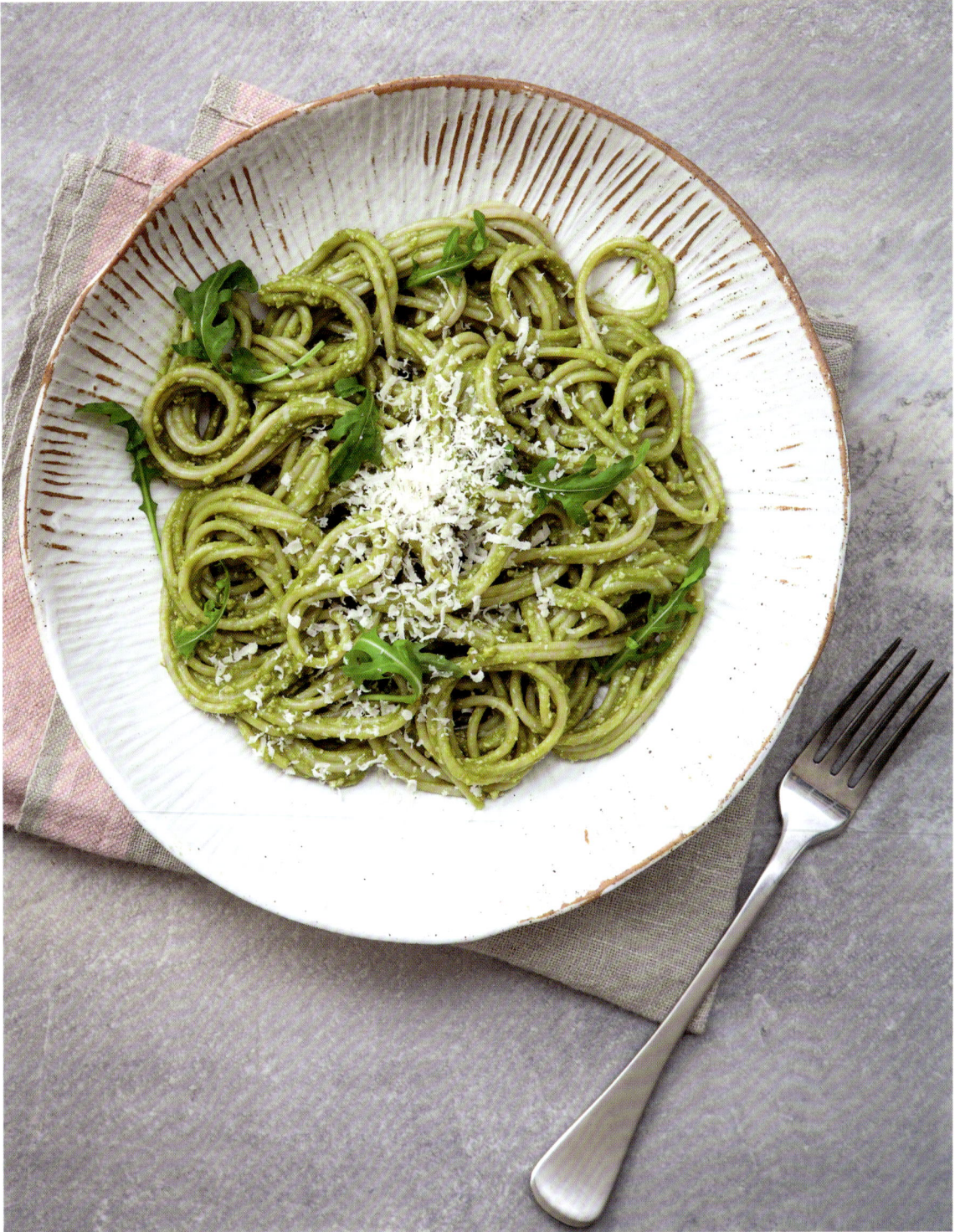

Black Bean Nut Roast

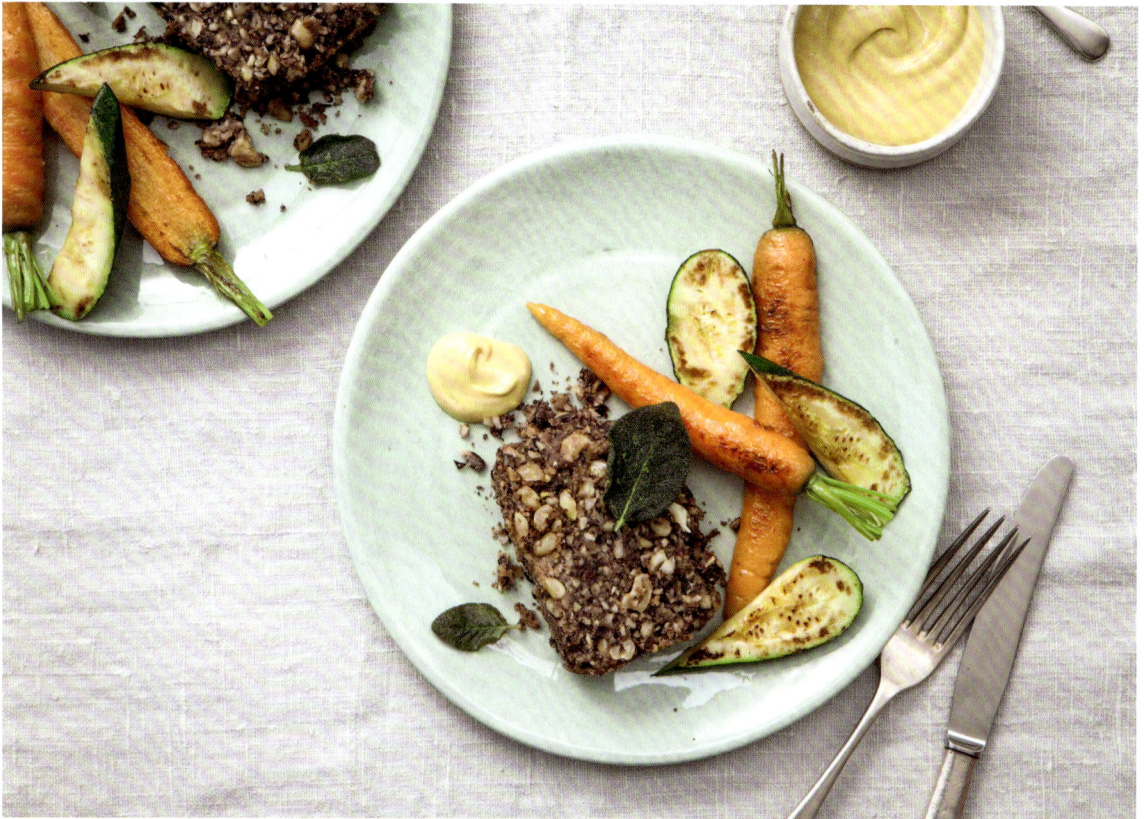

2 x 400g (14oz) cans black beans,
   rinsed and drained
125g (4½oz) pine nuts
150g (5½oz) cashew nuts
4 garlic cloves, crushed
4 sage leaves, chopped
50g (1¾oz) oats
1 tablespoon olive oil, plus extra
   for greasing
salt and black pepper

To serve:
roasted carrots
roasted courgettes
mustard
crispy fried sage leaves

Black beans are a great source of vegetarian protein. They are a slow-release carbohydrate due to their fibre content and are a great source of folate and magnesium.

1. Preheat the oven to 180°C (350°F), Gas Mark 4. Place all of the nut roast ingredients in a food processor and blitz until well mixed and fairly smooth. Transfer the mixture to a greased loaf tin and press down so it looks like a loaf of bread.

2. Cover with foil and cook for 30–35 minutes, then leave to rest for 15 minutes. Slice and serve with roasted carrots and courgettes, mustard and crispy fried sage leaves.

Bang Bang Chicken Salad

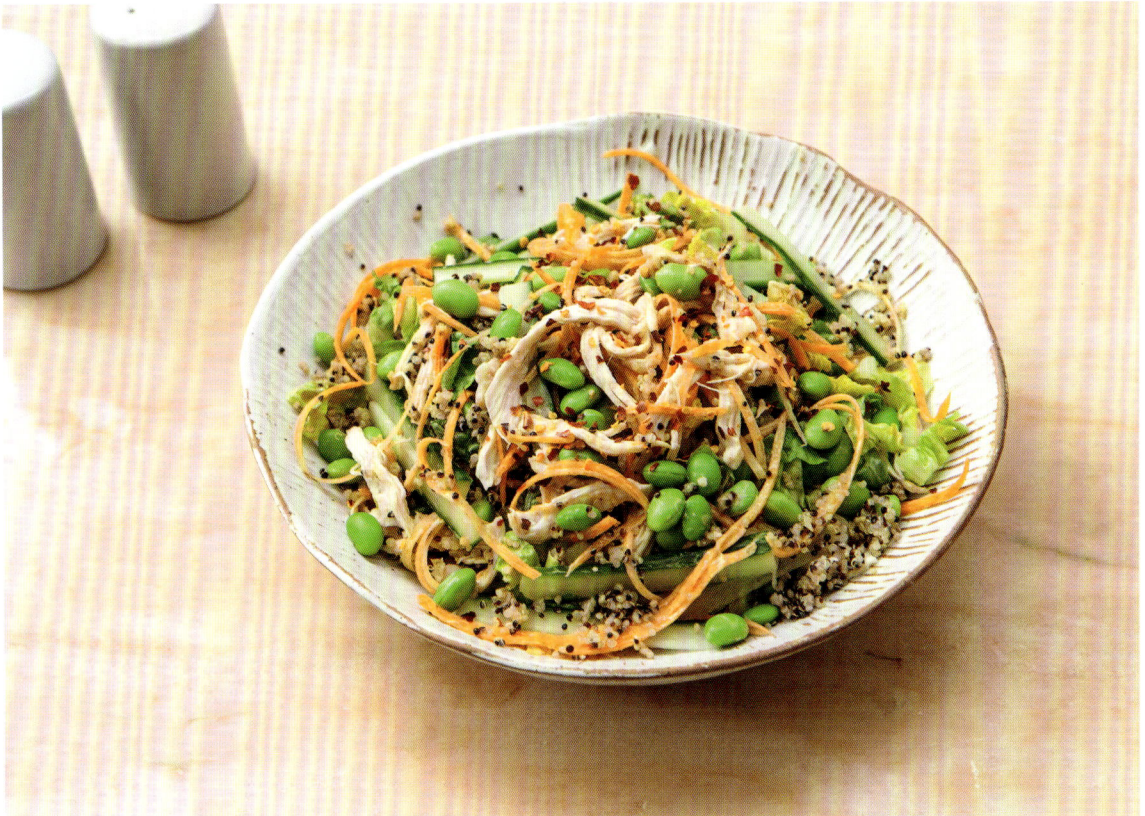

1 Little Gem lettuce, shredded
1 carrot, peeled and cut into
    matchsticks
½ cucumber, cut into matchsticks
handful of edamame beans
125g (4½oz) cooked quinoa
1 cooked chicken breast, shredded

For the dressing:
1 tablespoon smooth peanut butter
1 tablespoon sesame oil
1 teaspoon maple syrup
pinch of chilli flakes
juice of 1 lime

This hearty lunch is packed full of protein. I've added edamame beans because they have such a good nutritional profile. They are high in vitamin K and folate, which helps to convert carbohydrates into energy.

1. Place the dressing ingredients in a serving bowl and whisk to combine. Add all the salad ingredients and toss together, then serve.

All-in-One Chicken Tray Bake

Garlic is a wonderful food, as it helps to ward off colds and bacterial infections (try eating it raw if you are feeling especially run down or have a cough). This dish works equally well with halloumi or salmon instead of chicken.

Serves 2

1 sweet potato, diced
1 courgette, diced
1 red onion, sliced
1 yellow pepper, cored, deseeded
    and diced
handful of cherry tomatoes
3 small garlic cloves, skin on
2 tablespoons olive oil
1–2 tablespoons balsamic vinegar
2 chicken breasts
handful of basil leaves
salt and black pepper

1. Preheat the oven to 190°C (375°F), Gas Mark 5. Place the vegetables and garlic in a large roasting tin or ovenproof dish with the oil and vinegar. Make three deep cuts across the top of each chicken breast to help soak up the flavours, then place in the tin with the veggies. Season well, then toss thoroughly to make sure everything has been coated well in the oil and vinegar.

2. Cook for 35–40 minutes, or until the chicken is cooked through and the vegetables are golden brown. Carefully remove the garlic cloves and set aside to cool for a minute or two, then squeeze the flesh out of the skins. Return the garlic flesh to the tin with the basil and stir through the chicken and veggies. Finish with a good grinding of black pepper.

```
PREPARATION IS KEY

Success on this plan comes down to
preparation and organization.

Make sure you freeze leftovers and take
your meals and snacks with you when you
leave the house.

Get used to packing snacks in your bag
and popping meals in plastic containers
so that you never get caught out.
```

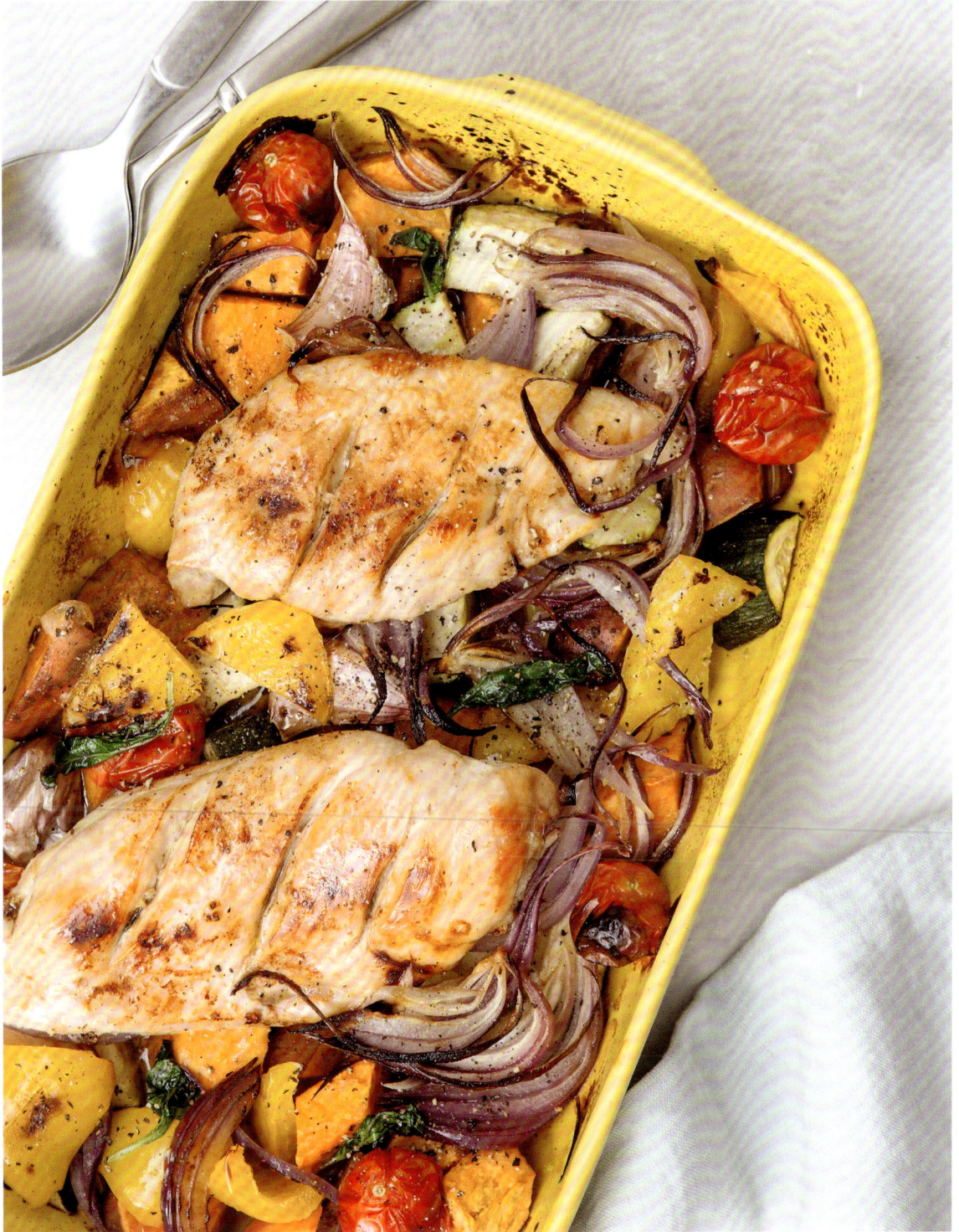

Creamy Chicken & Mash

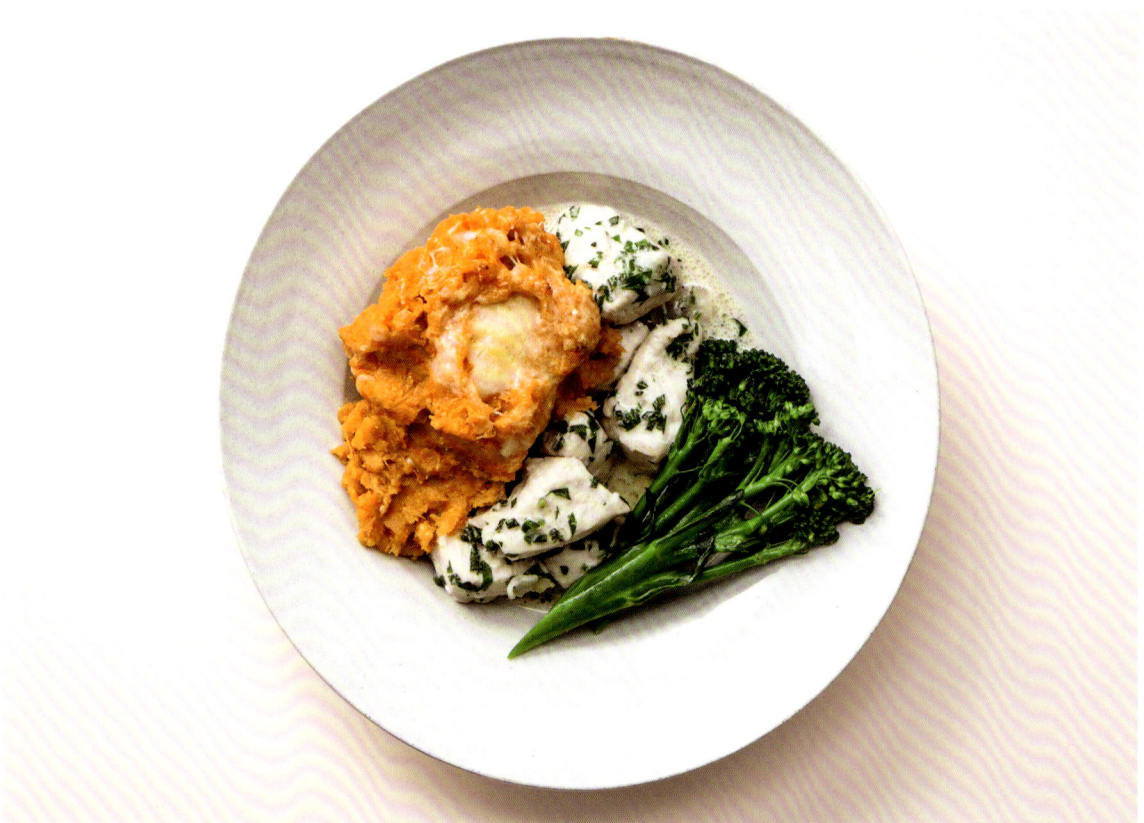

1 tablespoon olive oil
2 chicken breasts, cut into chunks
1 onion, chopped
1 garlic clove, crushed
400ml (14fl oz) coconut milk
handful of chopped parsley
1 sweet potato, diced
knob of butter
handful of grated Cheddar cheese
salt and black pepper
broccoli, to serve

I love this dish. It is hearty and comforting and packed with nutrients.

1. Heat the olive oil in a frying pan over a medium heat, add the chicken, onion and garlic and cook for 5–7 minutes, or until the onion has softened. Add the coconut milk, bring to the boil, then reduce the heat and simmer for 10 minutes, or until the sauce has thickened and the chicken is cooked through. Stir through the chopped parsley.

2. Meanwhile, cook the sweet potato in a saucepan of lightly salted boiling water for 10–15 minutes, or until completely tender. Drain and mash the potato with a knob of butter and season to taste.

3. Serve the chicken with the mashed sweet potato, sprinkled with grated cheese, and broccoli.

Mediterranean Chicken

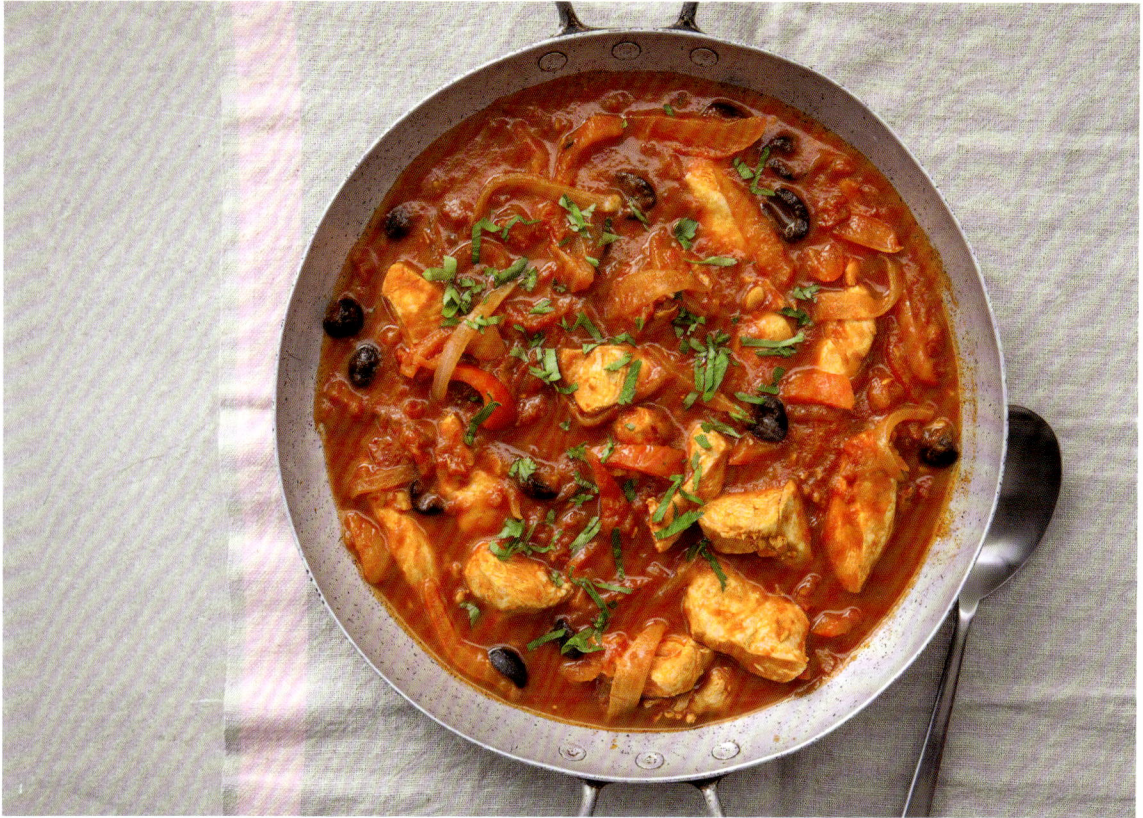

Serves 2

1 tablespoon olive oil
1 onion, sliced
1 red pepper, cored, deseeded
   and sliced
4 garlic cloves, finely chopped
1 tablespoon smoked paprika
1 teaspoon ground cumin
1 tablespoon tomato purée
400g (14oz) can chopped tomatoes
2 chicken breasts, cut into chunks
12 black olives, halved
salt and black pepper
chopped parsley, to garnish

This is a simple and delicious dish that's bursting with flavour. It contains cumin, which is high in antioxidants and has anti-inflammatory properties.

1. Heat the olive oil in a frying pan over a medium heat, add the onion and red pepper and cook for 5–7 minutes, or until softened. Add the garlic and cook for 1 minute more. Add the spices, tomato purée and chopped tomatoes and bring to the boil.

2. Add the chicken and olives, season to taste, reduce the heat and simmer for 20 minutes, or until the chicken is cooked through. Serve sprinkled with chopped parsley.

Chicken-stuffed Peppers with Ricotta & Harissa

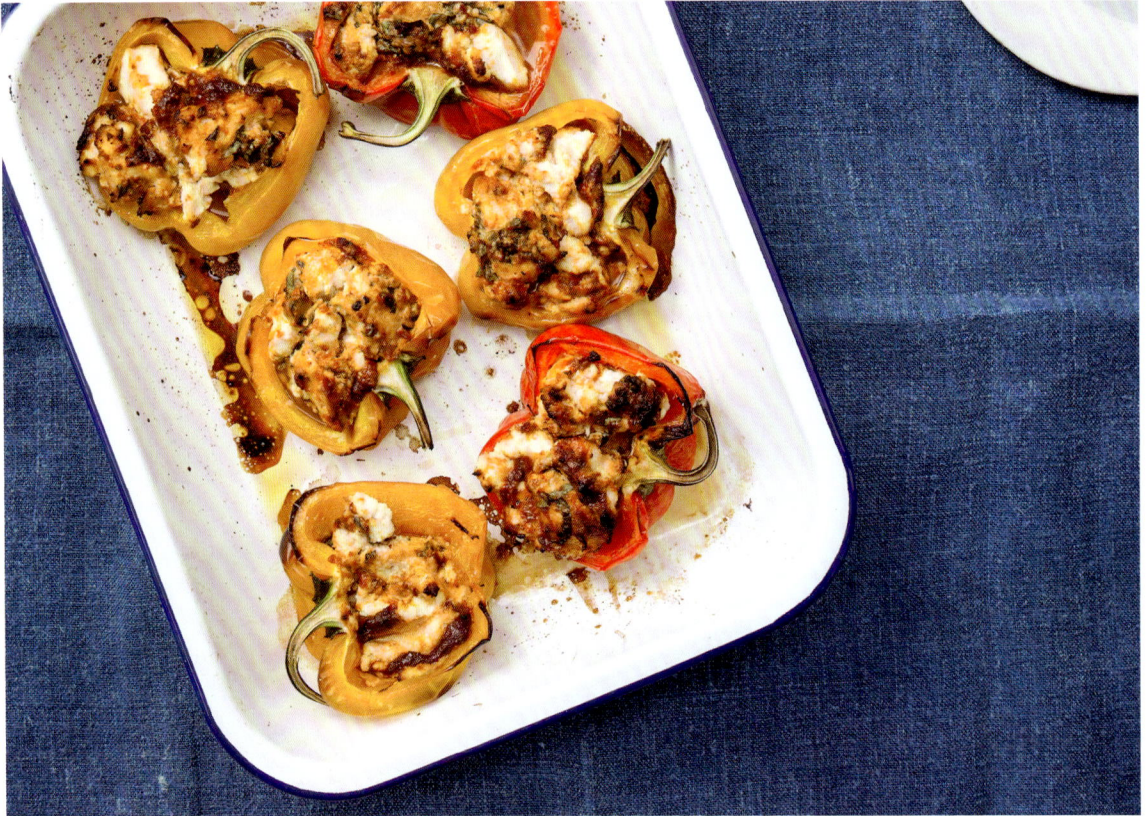

<u>Serves 2-3</u>

3 peppers
2 chicken breasts, diced
1 tablespoon ricotta
2 teaspoons harissa
handful of chopped basil
olive oil, for drizzling
salt and black pepper

To serve:
crisp green salad
roast or new potatoes

This is a really tasty dish. I've used chicken for protein and harissa for a bit of a kick. You can use turkey instead, or if you would prefer to make a vegetarian version, use rice or quinoa.

1. Preheat the oven to 190°C (375°F), Gas Mark 5. Slice the peppers in half and use a spoon to scoop out any seeds inside.

2. Place the chicken, ricotta, harissa and basil in a bowl, season well and lightly mix, trying to keep a bit of a ripple effect. Divide the mixture between the peppers.

3. Drizzle with a little olive oil and cook for 35–40 minutes, or until the peppers are turning golden and the chicken is cooked through. Serve with a crisp green salad and roast or new potatoes.

Bean Chilli with Sweet Potato

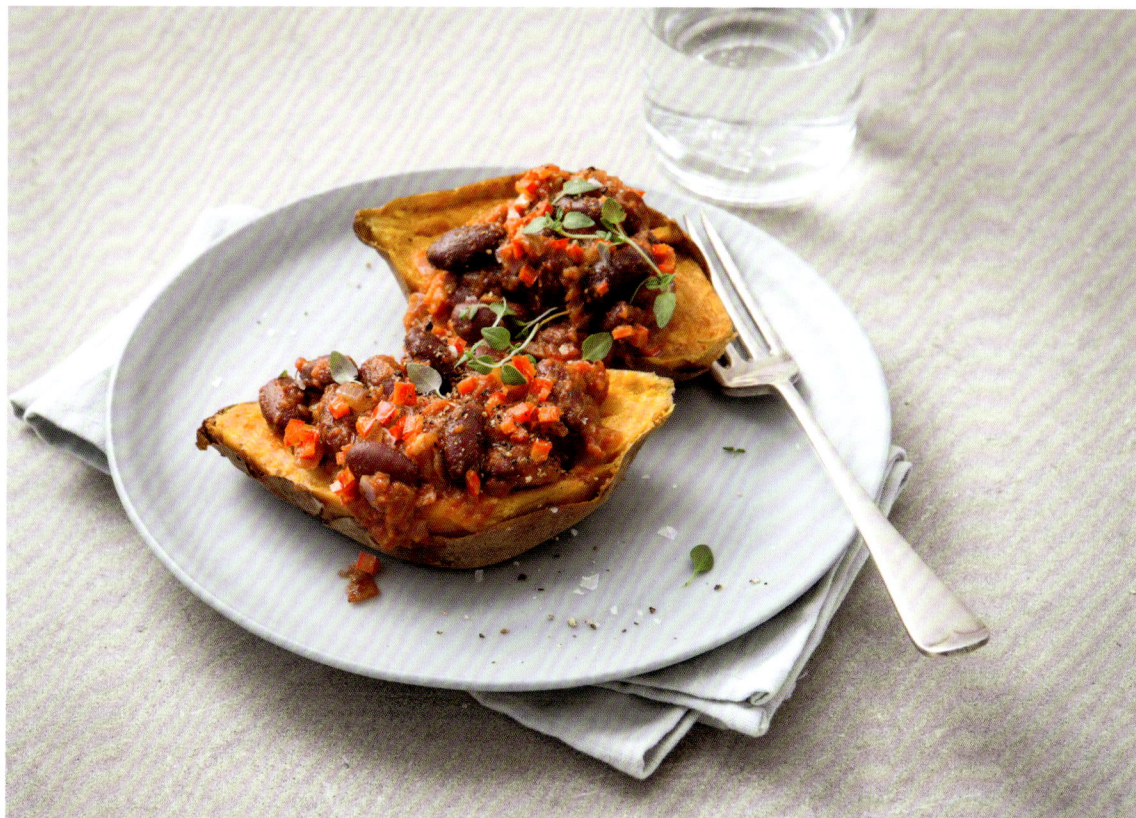

Serves 4

4 sweet potatoes
1 tablespoon olive oil
1 garlic clove, crushed
1 red onion, chopped
1 red chilli, deseeded and chopped
400g (14oz) can kidney beans, rinsed
    and drained
400g (14oz) can chopped tomatoes
3 tablespoons balsamic vinegar
1 thyme sprig, plus extra to garnish
salt and black pepper

I love sweet potatoes! They taste delicious and are much more nutrient-dense than white potatoes, containing higher amounts of vitamin C and B vitamins. They are also an excellent source of vitamin A.

1. Preheat the oven to 200°C (400°F), Gas Mark 6. Cook the sweet potatoes in their skins for 35–40 minutes, or until tender.

2. Meanwhile, heat the oil in a large saucepan, add the garlic, onion and chilli and cook for 5 minutes, or until softened. Add all the remaining ingredients, season to taste and bring to the boil. Reduce the heat and simmer for 15 minutes, or until thickened.

3. Spoon one-quarter of the bean chilli on top of each jacket potato and garnish with thyme. Any leftover chilli can be kept in an airtight container in the refrigerator for up to 5 days.

Beef & Broccoli Stir-fry

I've used beef in this stir-fry because it is an excellent source of iron. If you have low iron levels you will feel tired and out of breath just walking up the stairs. Beef is also a great source of zinc, which is needed to make all the hormones in your body, including cortisol.

<u>Serves 2</u>

1 tablespoon olive oil
250g (9oz) steak, sliced
350g (12oz) broccoli, cut into small florets
1 red onion, sliced
1 red pepper, cored, deseeded and sliced
handful of cashew nuts
salt and black pepper
brown rice, to serve

For the sauce
4 tablespoons soy sauce
2 tablespoons honey
1 teaspoon mustard
1 tablespoon sesame seeds

1. Heat the oil in a wok or large frying pan over a high heat, add the steak, veggies and nuts and stir-fry for 7–10 minutes, or until the veggies are tender.

2. Add the sauce ingredients and cook for another 2–3 minutes, stirring constantly. Serve immediately with brown rice.

THINGS THAT CAN MAKE YOUR ANXIETY WORSE:

Irregular sleep
Watching or reading a lot of negative news
Caffeine
Saying 'yes' to too many things
Stress and conflict
Too much social media
Isolating yourself

Look after yourself by trying to avoid these wherever possible.

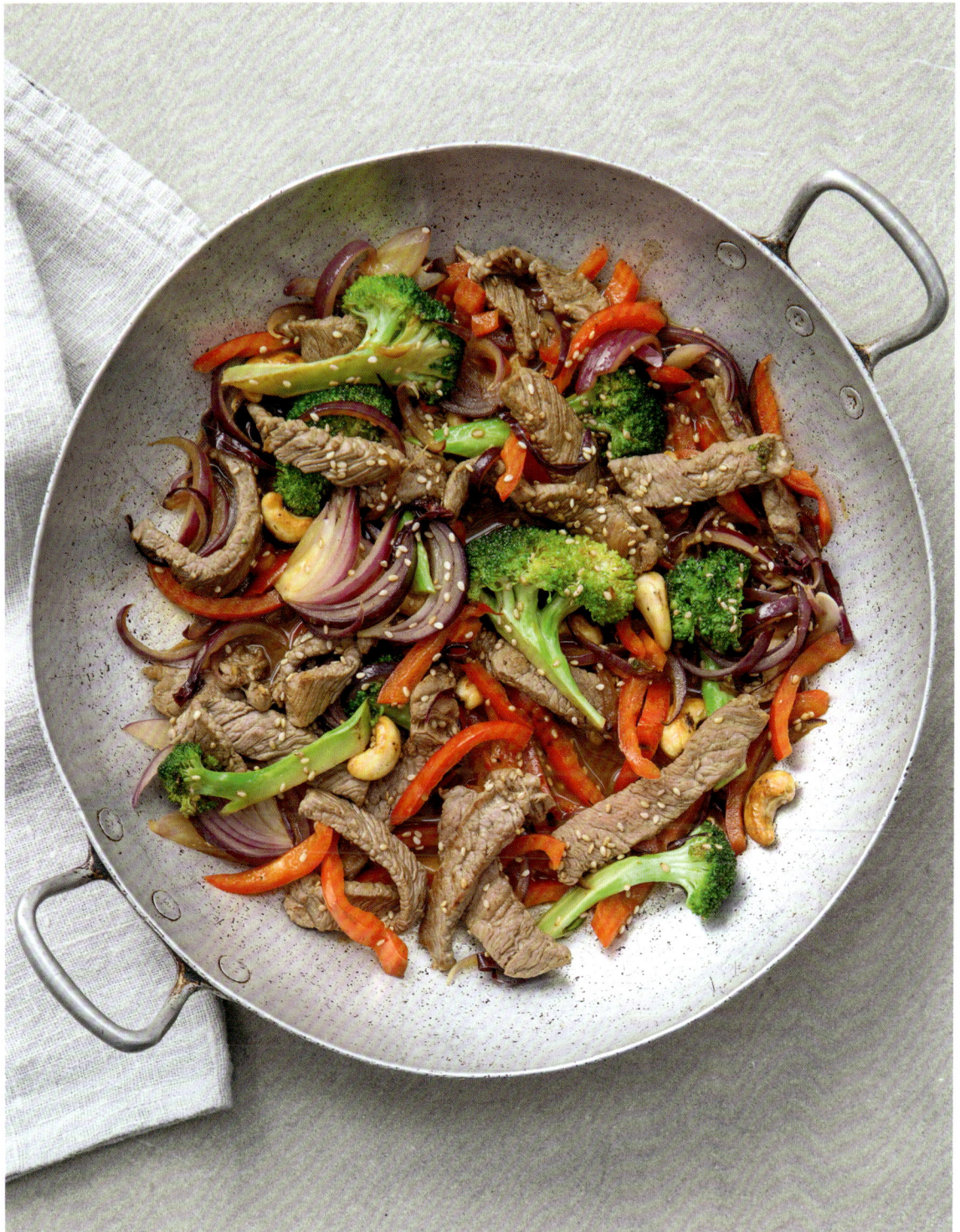

Creamy Beef Stew

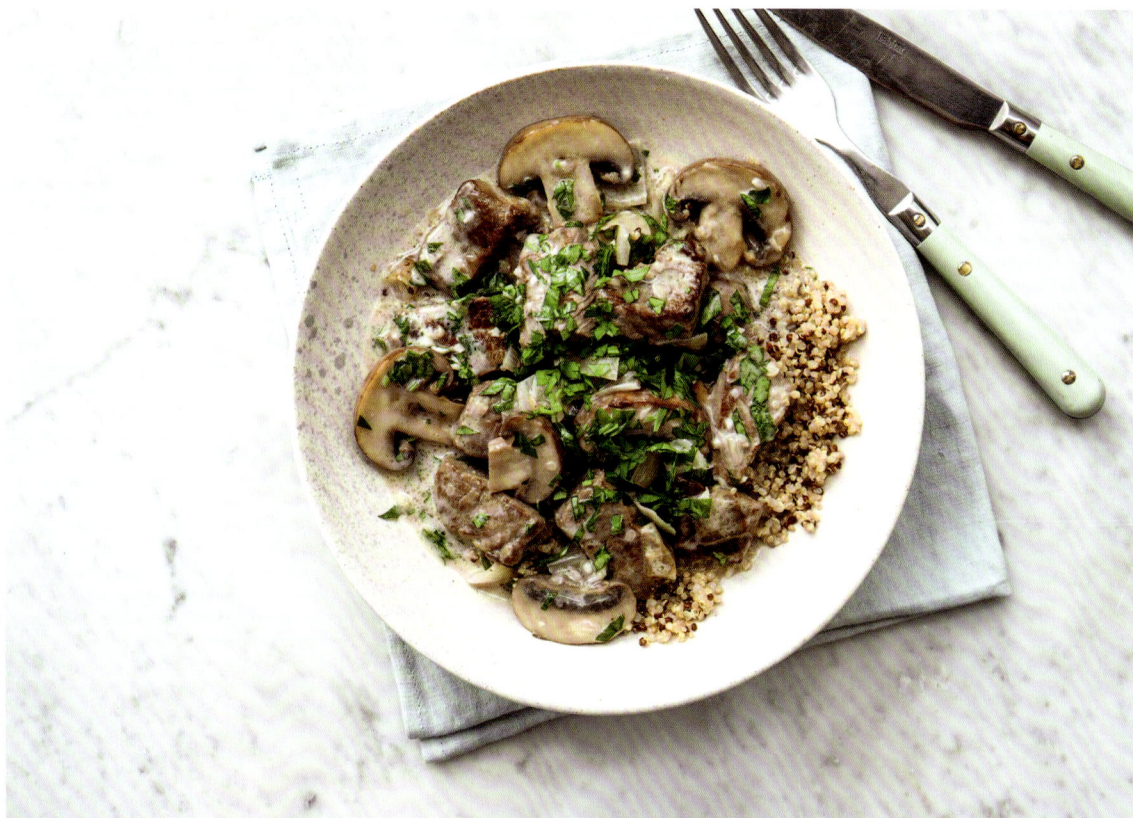

Serves 2

knob of butter
250g (9oz) beef, diced
1 onion, diced
100g (3½oz) mushrooms, sliced
2 garlic cloves, crushed
400ml (14fl oz) coconut milk
truffle oil, for drizzling
salt and black pepper
quinoa, to serve
small handful of chopped parsley,
    to garnish

This easy-to-make stew is absolutely delicious. You can use any type of mushroom – most mushrooms are good sources of fibre and contain B vitamins and selenium.

1. Heat the butter in a large saucepan or casserole over a medium-high heat, add the beef, onion, mushrooms and garlic and cook, stirring regularly, for 10 minutes.

2. Add the coconut milk, bring to the boil, then reduce the heat and simmer for 15 minutes, or until the sauce has thickened and the beef is tender. Season to taste, drizzle with truffle oil and serve on a bed of quinoa. Garnish with parsley.

Turkey Burgers

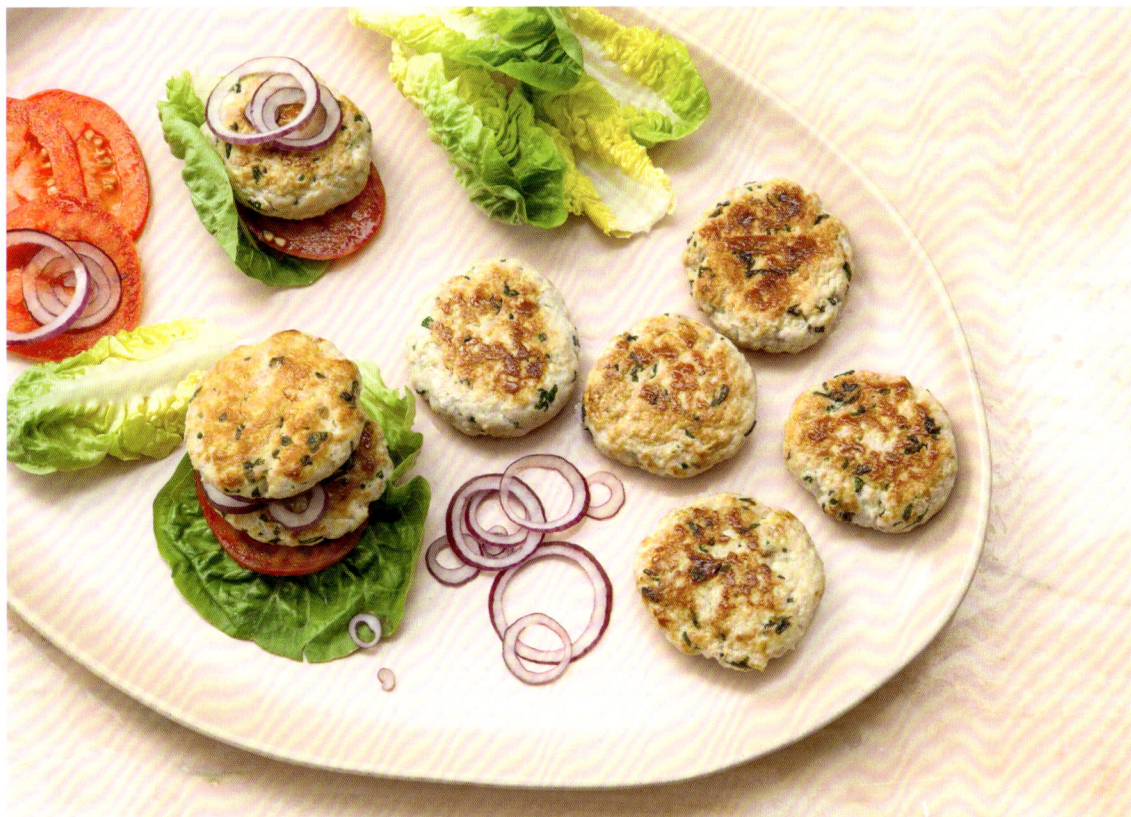

<u>Serves 3</u>

450g (1lb) minced turkey
½ ripe avocado, mashed
50g (1¾oz) Parmesan cheese, grated
handful of chopped basil leaves
1 tablespoon olive oil (optional)
salt and black pepper

To serve:
lettuce leaves
red onion slices
tomato slices
green salad

These turkey burgers are super quick to make and can be eaten as a main meal or later as a snack if you are on the go.

1. Place the turkey in a bowl, add the avocado, Parmesan and basil and season to taste. Mix well with your hands, then divide the mixture into 10 equal portions and use damp hands to shape into small burger patties.

2. Heat the oil in a large frying pan and cook the patties for about 8 minutes, turning once, or until golden on both sides and cooked through. Alternatively, cook the patties under a preheated hot grill.

3. Serve the patties stacked in lettuce leaves with slices of onion and tomato, with a large green salad on the side.

Your Six Week Meal Plan

My six-week meal plan will be your food bible for the next 42 days and will put everything that you have read in the theory text into practice. Every day your meals are laid out for you. All you have to do is follow the plan and the results will come. This meal plan is free from refined sugar, gluten, caffeine and alcohol, instead focusing on the foods that give you energy – lean proteins, quality fats, fibre and smart carbs.

This meal plan is not a starvation diet. I want you to eat five times a day, at the following times:

Breakfast: 7–9am
Snack: 10–11am
Lunch: 12–2pm
Snack: 3–4pm
Dinner: 6–7pm

If your blood pressure is low and you feel dizzy from time to time, have a large glass of filtered water with half a teaspoon of rock salt every morning when you wake up (see page 67).

Following the Plan

There is room for flexibility on this plan. For example, if your dinner option one day is salmon but you only have cod, that is okay. If you don't like courgettes but you love broccoli, then swap it. As long as you are following the plan and sticking to the principles, small changes are fine. What doesn't work is when you decide to skip breakfast, eat soup for lunch then grab a sandwich on the go and a coffee because you ran out of time.

No.

The key to success on this plan is preparation and organization. As long as you get the food in and prepare the meals, you should start to feel more energy by Day 5.

Snacks

I have not included snacks in the meal plan, but do eat them if you are hungry throughout the day.

For some people, a smoothie for breakfast is not enough to fill them up, so you can always have a snack as well.

Please then make sure you have a snack mid-morning and mid-afternoon – choose from the recipes on pages 126–31.

The Perfect Plate

For each meal, half your plate should contain colourful veggies, one quarter should be carbohydrates and the other quarter should be protein and fats.

Portion Size

The below list indicates how much of each ingredient you should be eating:

Vegetables and fruit – Baseball
Meat and poultry – Palm of your hand, excluding fingers
Fish – Cheque book
Sweet potato – Computer mouse
Dried fruit, nuts and seeds – Golf ball
Oil, butter, margarine – Thumb tip
Quinoa, rice, oats – A rounded handful

Each recipe in this book will tell you how many people it serves. Follow the recipes, and you will be eating the right amount of each ingredient.

But if you're ever unsure of quantities, such as how many vegetables to serve a dish with or how much meat to buy, use the above list as a guide.

To Do

1. Start the meal plan. Get organized by shopping for the first week and prep your meals day by day.

2. Write down everything you eat in one day, then add some notes about how you feel. Are you feeling tired, or more alert than usual? This will help you identify which foods are making you tired and which more energized. Keep a log of what is going on so you can monitor how you feel and your progress.

3. I also want you to keep track of your calories to make sure you are not undereating (see page 81).

Meal Planner—Week 1

	Breakfast	Lunch	Dinner
Monday	Fruity Quinoa Bowl (page 117)	Lentil Dahl with Roasted Garlic (page 159)	Beef & Broccoli Stir-fry (page 192)
Tuesday	Beetroot Smoothie (page 104)	Mexican Brown Rice Rainbow Bowl (page 138)	Quick Fish Stew with Olives & Lemon (page 179)
Wednesday	Sunshine Smoothie (page 110)	Simple Salmon Salad (page 143)	Puttanesca Prawn Pasta (page 171)
Thursday	Chocolate Peanut Smoothie (page 105)	Greek Pasta Salad with Quick Pickled Red Onions (page 136)	Grilled Fish Kebabs (page 176)
Friday	Black Beans & Avocado on Toast (page 121)	Raw Vegan Sushi (page 146)	Bean Chilli with Sweet Potato (page 191)
Saturday	Poached Eggs on Veggies (page 120)	Coconut, Vegetable & Chicken Soup (page 164)	Avocado Pesto Spaghetti (page 182)
Sunday	Banana & Mixed Berry Pancakes (page 118)	Courgette Fritters with Smoked Salmon (page 154)	Mediterranean Chicken (page 189)

Notes:

Meal Planner—Week 2

	Breakfast	Lunch	Dinner
Monday	Mango, Strawberry & Coconut Smoothie (page 108)	Mexican Brown Rice Rainbow Bowl (page 138)	Turkey & Aubergine Parmigiana (page 181)
Tuesday	Beetroot Hash with Eggs (page 122)	Avocado & Feta Pitta Pockets (page 158)	Prawn & Cashew Stir-fry (page 170)
Wednesday	Fresh Mint Smoothie (page 106)	Spanish Omelette with Sweet Potato & Onion (page 156)	Black Bean Nut Roast (page 184)
Thursday	Blueberry Smoothie (page 111)	Sesame Soba Noodle Salad (page 135)	Avocado Pesto Spaghetti (page 182)
Friday	Raspberry & Chia Seed Pudding (page 124)	Beetroot Soup (page 161)	Turkey Burgers (page 195)
Saturday	Chocolate Protein Smoothie (page 107)	Lentil Dahl with Roasted Garlic (page 159)	Pan-fried Cod with Mint Pea Mash (page 175)
Sunday	Poached Eggs on Veggies (page 120)	Mango, Chicken & Cashew Salad (page 150)	Roast Squash Quinoa Risotto (page 180)

Notes:

Meal Planner—Week 3

	Breakfast	Lunch	Dinner
Monday	Sunshine Smoothie (page 110)	Smoked Mackerel, Beetroot & Watercress Salad (page 140)	Creamy Chicken & Mash (page 188)
Tuesday	Beetroot Hash with Eggs (page 122)	Garlic & Ginger Carrot Soup (page 160)	Baked Salmon with Butter Bean Mash (page 172)
Wednesday	Vanilla Protein Smoothie (page 115)	Prawn & Courgette Bowl with Watercress Dressing (page 139)	Chicken-stuffed Peppers with Ricotta & Harissa (page 190)
Thursday	Raspberry & Chia Seed Pudding (page 124)	Broccoli & Turmeric Soup (page 162)	Turkey Burgers (page 195)
Friday	Pina Colada Smoothie (page 112)	Chickpea, Avocado & Feta Salad (page 137)	All-in-One Chicken Tray Bake (page 186)
Saturday	Black Beans & Avocado on Toast (page 121)	Salmon & Pear Salad (page 144)	Puttanesca Prawn Pasta (page 171)
Sunday	Blue Spirulina Smoothie (page 113)	Glow Bowl (page 134)	Creamy Beef Stew (page 194)

Notes:

Meal Planner—Week 4

	Breakfast	Lunch	Dinner
Monday	Raspberry Coconut Smoothie (page 114)	Prawn & Corn Salad (page 142)	Bang Bang Chicken Salad (page 185)
Tuesday	Fruity Quinoa Bowl (page 117)	Seared Tuna Wraps with Matcha Dip (page 147)	Avocado Pesto Spaghetti (page 182)
Wednesday	Mango, Strawberry & Coconut Smoothie (page 108)	Chicken & Avocado Cabbage Wraps (page 153)	Bean Chilli with Sweet Potato (page 191)
Thursday	Banana & Mixed Berry Pancakes (page 118)	Steamed Pesto Salmon with Green Salad (page 152)	Chicken-stuffed Peppers with Ricotta & Harissa (page 190)
Friday	Power Smoothie (page 116)	Mexican Brown Rice Rainbow Bowl (page 138)	Smoked Mackerel Layer Bake (page 169)
Saturday	Poached Eggs on Veggies (page 120)	Spanish Omelette with Sweet Potato & Onion (page 156)	Steamed Ginger & Soy Fish Parcels (page 174)
Sunday	Raspberry Coconut Smoothie (page 114)	Chickpea, Avocado & Feta Salad (page 137)	Prawn & Cashew Stir-fry (page 170)

Notes:

_____

_____

_____

_____

_____

_____

Meal Planner—Week 5

	Breakfast	Lunch	Dinner
Monday	Poached Eggs on Veggies (page 120)	Raw Vegan Sushi (page 146)	Salmon Fishcakes (page 178)
Tuesday	Vanilla Protein Smoothie (page 115)	Avocado & Feta Pitta Pockets (page 158)	Bang Bang Chicken Salad (page 185)
Wednesday	Fruity Quinoa Bowl (page 117)	Beetroot Falafel with Green Quinoa Salad (page 148)	Sweet Sea Bass Salad (page 168)
Thursday	Raspberry & Chia Seed Pudding (page 124)	Chickpea, Avocado & Feta Salad (page 137)	Mediterranean Chicken (page 189)
Friday	Black Beans & Avocado on Toast (page 121)	Beetroot Soup (page 161)	Pan-fried Cod with Mint Pea Mash (page 175)
Saturday	Blueberry Smoothie (page 111)	Greek Pasta Salad with Quick Pickled Red Onions (page 136)	Beef & Broccoli Stir-fry (page 192)
Sunday	Blue Spirulina Smoothie (page 113)	Salmon & Pear Salad (page 144)	Black Bean Nut Roast (page 184)

Notes:

_____

_____

_____

_____

_____

_____

_____

Meal Planner—Week 6

	Breakfast	**Lunch**	**Dinner**
Monday	Beetroot Smoothie (page 104)	Spanish Omelette with Sweet Potato & Onion (page 156)	Turkey Burgers (page 195)
Tuesday	Fruity Quinoa Bowl (page 117)	Smoked Mackerel, Beetroot & Watercress Salad (page 140)	All-in-One Chicken Tray Bake (page 186)
Wednesday	Coconut & Cranberry Energy Bars (page 128)	Prawn & Corn Salad (page 142)	Creamy Chicken & Mash (page 188)
Thursday	Sunshine Smoothie (page 110)	Beetroot Falafel with Green Quinoa Salad (page 148)	Quick Fish Stew with Olives & Lemon (page 179)
Friday	Beetroot Hash with Eggs (page 122)	Roasted Tomato & Basil Soup (page 165)	Baked Salmon with Butter Bean Mash (page 172)
Saturday	Poached Eggs on Veggies (page 120)	Chicken & Avocado Cabbage Wraps (page 153)	Roast Squash Quinoa Risotto (page 180)
Sunday	Banana & Mixed Berry Pancakes (page 118)	Sesame Soba Noodle Salad (page 135)	Prawn & Cashew Stir-fry (page 170)

Notes:

_____

_____

_____

_____

_____

_____

Glossary

References

Page 30 Healthy Safety Executive, 'Work-related stress, anxiety or depression statistics in Great Britain, 2019'

Page 49 Moncrieff, J., Cooper, R.E., Stockmann, T. *et al.*, 'The serotonin theory of depression: a systematic umbrella review of the evidence,' *Molecular Psychiatry,* 28, August 2023, pp.3243–3256

Berk, M., Williams, L.J., Jacka, F.N. *et al.*, 'So depression is an inflammatory disease, but where does the inflammation come from?,' *BMC Medicine,* 11, September 2013

Smith, R.S., *Cytokines and Depression: How Your Immune System Causes Depression,* 2010

Page 50 Winston, P.A., Hardwick, E. and Jaberi, N., 'Neuropsychiatric effects of caffeine', *Advances in Psychiatric Treatment,* 11(6), November 2005, 432–9

Page 51 Li, J., Wang, J., Wang, M., Zheng, L., Cen, Q., Wang, F., Zhu, L., Pang, R. and Zhang, A. '*Bifidobacterium*: a probiotic for the prevention and treatment of depression', *Front Microbiol*, May 2023

Ferrari, S., Mulè, S., Parini, F., Galla, R., Ruga, S., Rosso, G., Brovero, A., Molinari, C. and Uberti, F., 'The influence of the gut-brain axis on anxiety and depression: A review of the literature on the use of probiotics', *Journal of Traditional and Complementary Medicine*, 14(3), May 2024, pp.237–255

Page 52 Czaja-Bulsa, G., 'Non coeliac gluten sensitivity – A new disease with gluten intolerance', *Clinical Nutrition,* 34(2), April 2015, pp.189–94

Page 54 Genetics Home Reference, 'Your Guide to Understanding Genetic Conditions', Lactose Intolerance, https://ghr.nlm.nih.gov/condition/lactose-intolerance#statistics (accessed 17 January 2020)

Page 61 NHS, 'B vitamins and folic acid' www.nhs.uk/conditions/vitamins-and-minerals/vitamin-b/ (accessed 9 January 2020)

Page 62 Penckofer, S., Kouba, J., Byrn, M. and Estwing Ferrans, C., 'Vitamin D and Depression: Where is all the Sunshine?', *Issues in Mental Health Nursing*, 31(6), June 2010, pp.385–93

Page 68 Rhee, D.K. and Lee, S., 'Effects of ginseng on stress-related depression, anxiety, and the hypothalamic-pituitary-adrenal axis', *Journal of Ginseng Research*, 41(4), October 2017, pp.589–94

Page 76 Rodenbeck, A. and Hajak, G., 'Neuroendocrine dysregulation in primary insomnia', *Revue Neurologique*, 157(11 Pt 2), November 2001, pp57–61

Chang, A., Aeschbach, D., Duffy, J.F. and Czeisler, C.A., 'Evening use of light-emitting eReaders negatively affects sleep, circadian timing, and next-morning alertness', *Proceedings of the National Academy of Sciences*, 112(4), January 2015, pp.1232–7

Page 78 Okamoto-Mizuno, K., Mizuno, K., 'Effects of thermal environment on sleep and circadian rhythm', *Journal of Physiological Anthropology*, 31 (14), May 2012

Page 96 Black, D.S., O'Reilly, G.A., Olmstead, R. et al, 'Mindfulness Meditation and Improvement in Sleep Quality and Daytime Impairment Among Older Adults With Sleep Disturbances: A Randomized Clinical Trial', *JAMA Internal Medicine*, 175(4), April 2015, pp.494–501

Index

Acknowledgements

If you had told me, when I was lying in bed unable to lift my head off the pillow because I was so fatigued, that I'd write a book about my journey to recovery, I never would have believed you. But here we are!

My recovery would not have been possible without my twin sister Susie. She was my lifeline in the dark years that preceded my collapse. So I dedicate this book to her. Thank you Susie for being my saviour. You were always there when I needed you the most. I wouldn't be where I am today without you.

This book would not have been possible without my mentors and coaches along the way. I thank them for encouraging me to keep going and for always motivating me to spread my message and never give up. Their words of encouragement brought me back to life again.

I would also like to say a tremendous thank you to the team at Octopus, who have worked tirelessly to get this book looking as beautiful as it does. The time and dedication you've put into this whole project has astonished me.

I'd also like to thank Morwenna Loughman for helping me with a few of the recipes. It would have been much more challenging without your input!

And lastly I'd like to thank you, dear reader. You have shown me unexpected floods of support throughout my journey. Never have I felt so loved, supported and humbled.

Rosie xxx